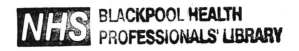

Get Through

MRCGP: Written Paper Module

I dedicate this book to Dr Jane Logan MRCGP
(my mentor, GP trainer and senior GP Principal)

Get Through
MRCGP: Written Paper Module

Una Coales MD FRCS FRCSOto DRCOG DFFP MRCGP
GP, London, UK

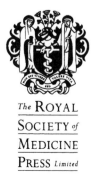

The ROYAL
SOCIETY of
MEDICINE
PRESS Limited

© 2005 Royal Society of Medicine Press Ltd

Reprinted 2006 (twice)

Published by the Royal Society of Medicine Press Ltd
1 Wimpole Street, London W1G 0AE, UK
Tel: +44 (0)20 7290 2921
Fax: +44 (0)20 7290 2929
Email: publishing@rsm.ac.uk
Website: www.rsmpress.co.uk

British Library Cataloguing in Publication Data
A catalogue record for this book is available from the British Library

ISBN 1-85315-621-3

Distribution in Europe and Rest of World:
Marston Book Services Ltd
PO Box 269
Abingdon
Oxon OX14 4YN, UK
Tel: +44 (0)1235 465500
Fax: +44 (0)1235 465555
Email: direct.order@marston.co.uk

Distribution in the USA and Canada:
Royal Society of Medicine Press Ltd
c/o Jamco Distribution Inc
1401 Lakeway Drive
Lewisville, TX 75057, USA
Tel: +1 800 538 1287
Fax: +1 972 353 1303
Email: jamco@majors.com

Distribution in Australia and New Zealand:
Elsevier Australia
30-52 Smidmore Street
Marrikville NSW 2204, Australia
Tel: +61 2 9349 5811
Fax: +61 2 9349 5911
Email: service@elsevier.com.au

Typeset by Phoenix Photosetting, Chatham, Kent
Printed and bound in Great Britain by Bell & Bain Ltd, Glasgow

Contents

Preface

This book accompanies my *Get Through MRCGP: New MCQ Module*, *Get Through MRCGP: Oral and Video Modules*, and *Get Through MRCGP: Hot Topics* series. It contains five sample papers for the MRCGP written module with each paper comprising 12 essay questions. Running my MRCGP course in London has made me aware that many candidates do not know how to structure their answers for the written paper. The Royal College of General Practitioners offers sample past written questions and examiners' comments on their website but does not give practical examples of how to answer the papers. This book gives you a structured guide to answering these questions and offers you practice on papers that are similar to past exam papers. Reference sources include the weekly *British Medical Journal*, weekly *Doctor* and *GP* magazines, *The Oxford Handbook Series*, the BNF, *Clinical Evidence*, and websites for current government and royal college guidelines.

Una Coales
January 2005
ufcmd@aol.com

Recommended Texts and References

Birtwhistle J, *et al*. *Oxford Handbook of General Practice*. Oxford: Oxford University Press, Oxford, 2002.

Clinical Evidence. London: BMJ Publishing Group.

Coales U. *Get Through MRCGP: Hot Topics*. London: Royal Society of Medicine Press, London, 2005.

Coales U. *Get Through MRCGP: New MCQ Module*. London: Royal Society of Medicine Press, 2003.

Coales U. *Get Through MRCGP: Oral and Video Modules*. London: Royal Society of Medicine Press, 2004.

Collier JAB, *et al*. *Oxford Handbook of Clinical Specialties*, 6th edn. Oxford: Oxford University Press, 2003.

Davies T, *et al*. *ABC of Mental Health*. London: BMJ Books, 1998.

Department of Health. *Drug Misuse and Dependence – Guidelines on Clinical Management*. London: HMSO, 1999.

Glasier A, *et al*. *Handbook of Family Planning and Reproductive Healthcare*, 4th edn. London: Churchill Livingstone, 2000.

Hope RA, *et al*. *Oxford Handbook of Clinical Medicine*, 5th edn. Oxford: Oxford University Press, 2001.

McLatchie GR. *Oxford Handbook of Clinical Surgery*, 2nd edn. Oxford: Oxford University Press, 2001.

Neighhbour R. *The Inner Consultation*. Berkshire: Librapharm, 2002.

Palmer KT. *Notes for the MRCGP*, 3rd edn. Oxford: Blackwell Science Ltd, 2001.

Royal Pharmaceutical Society of Great Britain. *British National Formulary*. London: British Medical Association, 2004.

Handy Tips for the MRCGP Written Paper Module

The written paper module consists of 12 essay questions. At least 3 of the 12 questions will ask you to *critically appraise a paper*, so the overall paper is extended to 3.5 hours to accommodate 30 minutes of reading time. I have included an outline of what you should include in your short answers (preferably in outline format with headings underlined). I have supplied you with my own set of mnemonics to remember lists but feel free to improvise.

At least 6 of the 12 written papers will ask you to *discuss issues*. Under issues, I have given you an outline of what you should cover in your short answers. These buzz words will apply no matter what the core subject heading!

The written paper may include a question on *screening programmes*. I have included an outline using Wilson and Jungner's criteria. Alternatively, the written paper may ask you to come up with a *protocol* and I have included an appropriate outline to use for this.

Two of the 12 papers will ask you to cite evidence-based medicine on various clinical topics. Short of reading every weekly *BMJ* and monthly *BJGP* from the previous year, familiarise yourself with *BMJ* review articles/trials/NSF guidelines/clinical evidence in hot topic areas. As a GP registrar, you can join the Royal College of General Practitioners as an associate member and receive the monthly *BJGP* for free.

Read the contents page and highlight interesting hot topics. You will not be expected to cite chapter and verse, but if you can mention basic principles, and list anything and everything you have read—journals, textbooks, lectures, etc, you will be able to fill in the empty spaces. Do not leave blank spaces.

For merit, you must quote one paper per essay question. For instance, quote the Russell paper that says that 5% of patients will listen to a doctor's advice on stopping smoking if brief advice is offered, or that spending 1 minute of the 10 minute consultation on health promotion can make a difference (Wilson A, McDonald P, Hayes L, Cooney J. Health Promotion in the general practice consultation: a minute makes a difference. *BMJ* 1992 Jan;304:227–230). Remember to mention the journal, month and year of publication. Note that it will be a different examiner marking each question, so by all means repeat yourself.

I have also included a list of papers to quote for the various Hot Topics so please commit a few trials and papers to memory and update the list regularly.

This book gives you five practice papers. You will recognise the style. It is similar to that used in the oral module. Once you have mastered all the papers in this book, you are ready to breeze through the written paper module. Good luck!

Critical Reading Protocol (mnemonic—IMROD)

1. Introduction (TBOAR)
    *   Title, author, institute (English, foreign), journal (respectable, peer reviewed)
    *   Background (to study)
    *   Originality (idea behind the study)
    *   Aims (clearly stated). Does the study match up to the aims?
    *   Relevance (to general practice)

2. Methods (DOS)
    *   Design (longitudinal/cross-sectional, observational/experimental, qualitative/quantitative, retrospective/prospective) $AICS$.
        — Is the study design appropriate? Repeatable?
        — Are the instruments and questionnaires reliable (same result if repeated) and validated (answers the research question)?
        — Are the confounding variables dealt with?
        — Is there a gold standard for comparison?
    *   Outcome measures (criteria appropriate/clearly defined?)
        — Are the end-points soft or hard and appropriate?
        — all the relevant outcomes included?
        — Is it truly blind to clinicians and patients?
    *   Subjects (inclusion and exclusion criteria clear?)
        — Are they representative of the population in question? Are they similar in age, sex, ethnic distribution and socioeconomic class?
        — Were controls used? Was the use of controls appropriate?
        — Was the selection of subjects and controls without bias?
        — Is the sample size sufficient to detect significant statistical results?
        — Has the power been calculated?
        — Has the sample been unchanged?
        — Does the method of randomisation allow reproduction of the experiment?

— Is the treatment plan clear?

— Has the time span been defined and is it appropriate?

3. Results (TURDS)
   - Tables and graphs. Understandable and clear. Are the data represented accurately?
   - Response rate reasonable (>70%)?
   - Dropouts—have the characteristics of the dropouts (failure to respond, non-attenders) been defined? Are all the subjects accounted for?
   - Statistics—is the statistical analysis used clear and appropriate for the design of the study? Does it include confidence limits and is the p value <0.05?

4. Discussion (CACA)
   - Critical evaluation of results—have the results been discussed with respect to other literature or compared to prior research? Have the applicability and limitations been discussed?
   - Aims—met?
   - Conclusions—consistent with results, justified with realistic speculations?
   - Applicability—to your population. Is it likely to change your practice?

5. Others (CORE)
   - Conflicts of interest—acknowledged source of funding (pharmaceutical)?
   - Overall—clear, ethical, valid, worthwhile study. Are conclusions affordable, available and sensible for your practice?
   - References—current?
   - Ethics—local ethical committee approval?

Relevant Issues: Topics to be Covered

1. Issues for the doctor (mnemonic—SHIP DRS COMMUNICATIONS)
   - Self-esteem
   - Health assessment
   - Input
   - Pressure to prescribe
   - Dependency
   - Record keeping
   - Sympathy
   - Constraints of time/chaperone
   - Opportunistic health promotion
   - Managing presenting problem
   - Moral code
   - Up-to-date practice
   - Non-judgmental care/gate-keeping
   - Investigations
   - Consent/confidentiality
   - Active listening/appraisal
   - Transcultural conflict
   - Irritation of patient
   - Open questioning
   - Need to justify actions
   - Shared care/referral

2. Issues for the patient (mnemonic—ABCD SPACESHIP)
   - Awareness of danger
   - Beliefs
   - Chronic disease/cultural
   - Denial
   - Stress
   - Peer pressure
   - Autonomy
   - Concern
   - Embarrassment/expectations

- Social support
- Hidden agenda
- Issues deeper
- Physical complaint

3. Issues for the practice (mnemonic—GRASP ALLOWANCES)
   - Guidelines
   - Review
   - Audit
   - Staff
   - Practice formulary/partnership dynamics/practice development plan
   - Available rooms
   - Local services
   - Locums
   - Open access
   - Written policies
   - Agreed practice policy
   - Nurses/nurse practitioners
   - Costs of administration/changes to existing system
   - Ease of availability
   - Safety issues for building/handicapped access

4. Legal and ethical issues
   - Personal ethics
   - Age of consent
   - Informed consent
   - Consult with your defence union/GMC/BMA
   - DVLA
   - Duty of confidentiality
   - Legal test of competency

5. Treatment issues
   - Comprehensive record keeping
   - Follow-up regime
   - Awareness of side-effects
   - Mutual agreement on therapeutic approach
   - Address fears
   - Implications of long-term therapy
   - Lifestyle advice
   - Community treatment

- Medical monitoring of drug levels
- Non-drug *vs* drug management
- Supportive role
- Ongoing education
- Crisis intervention
- Risks
- Share monitoring
- Committee on the Safety of Medicines

6. Wider issues
- Local support groups
- Availability of government resources
- Cost-benefit
- Refer to colleague if help needed
- Awareness of new treatments
- Making the practice adolescent-friendly
- Increased elderly coverage/demographics
- PCT
- Green paper to cut down on sick time
- NHS plan
- New GMS contract
- NSF guidelines/NICE
- Political—revalidation/rationing/recruitment/retention of doctors

7. Review, audit and follow-up
- Audit
- Failsafes/safety-netting
- Regular assessments
- Risk assessments
- Complaints
- Critical incidents

Requirements for Setting Up a Screening Programme or Protocol

Wilson and Jungner's screening programme

Requirements (mnemonic—IATROGENIC)
- Important condition
- Acceptable treatment for this disease
- Treatment and diagnostic facilities available
- Recognisable latent and early symptomatic stage
- Opinions on who to treat are agreed
- Guaranteed safety and reliability of test
- Examination acceptable to patient
- Natural history of disease is known
- Inexpensive and simple test
- Continuous rolling programme to be repeated at intervals

Protocol

The following points should be addressed in your discussion paper:

- Aims clearly stated
- Background—guidelines and protocols should be evidence-based
- Diagnosis should be clear
- Follow-up
- Audit performed regularly
- Responsibility for administrating or updating
- Refer—when to make urgent and routine referrals; exclusion criteria
- Review and update
- Target group

Relevant Papers/Trials

- 5% of patients will listen to doctors about quitting smoking if brief (2 mins) advice is offered (Russell MA *et al*, BMJ 1979;2:231).

Alcoholism

- Alcohol intervention in primary care (Kaner EF *et al*, *BJGP* 2001;51:822)—audit GPs identified 4000 risk drinkers but only 50% received brief intervention.

Alzheimer's disease (past paper topic)

- NICE recommendations to the NHS acknowledge the absence of satisfactory research on drugs for Alzheimer's disease (AD). Anticholinergic drugs for AD show evidence of clinical benefit that could be enough to secure approval despite lack of adequate means of measuring that benefit, no evidence of quality of life, and uninterpretable health economics.
- New drugs for AD and other dementias. (Bullock R, *Br J Psychiatry* 2002;180:135) CEI (cholinesterase inhibitors)—donepezil and vitamin E good evidence. CEI show initial cognitive and functional benefits but these wane as disease progresses. Symptomatic tx exists for AD.
- Cochrane database: Brown Univ Med School—statins ↓ risk of AD.
- Buxbaum JD *et al*, *Front Biosci* 2002;7:a50. Lovastatin decreases Alz beta-amyloid peptide in patients; delays onset and/or slows progression of AD.
- Pearson VE, *Ann Pharmacother* 2001;35:1406. Johns Hopkins Hospital—galantamine: a new Alzheimer's drug with a past life; acts as an acetylcholinesterase inhibitor and cholinergic nicotinic R agonist effective for mild-to-moderate AD symptoms.

Back pain (past paper topic)

- Clinical guidelines for the management of acute LBP (RCGP 1999).
- Systematic reviews of bedrest and advice to stay active for acute LBP (Waddell G *et al*, *BJGP* 1997;47:647).
- Predicting the outcome of sciatica at short-term follow-up (Vroomen PC *et al*, *BJGP* 2002;52:119).

Benign prostate hypertrophy (past paper topic)

- Uncertainty of PSA underlines need for *shared decision making*.
- Watchful waiting.
- Symptoms scoring, rectal, uroflowmetry, U/S, PSA. Need to consider sensitivity, specificity, PPV, and NPV. Discuss degree of benefits and harm from treatment options.
- Regional variations to treatment modalities.

Carers (past paper topic)

- Informal carers and the PCT (Simon C *et al*, *BJGP* 2001;51:655).
- Patient and carer satisfaction with Hospital at Home (Wilson A *et al*, *BJGP* 2002;52:9).

Cardiovascular risk factors

- Measurement and management of cardiovascular risk factors – is screening worthwhile? (McEwen SR *et al*, *Scot Med J* 1989;34:387).
- Framingham Heart Study —assessed RFs in a middle-aged pop in the USA and studied fatal + NF coronary events.
- CV RFs and disease in general practice (results of Nijmegen Cohort Study; Bakx JC *et al*, *BJGP* 2002;52:135 —7092 males RF age, smoking, serum chol $\geq$5.8 mmol/L, > 140/80 BP, BMI $\geq$27 kg/m^2, FHx of CVD, RR 1.8 for CVD morbidity for men and 1.7 for women with HTN).

Cervical cancer screening

- Cancer prevention in primary care. Screening for cervical cancer (Austoker J, *BMJ* 1994;309:517).

Chlamydia (past paper topic)

- *Chlamydia trachomatis*: opportunistic screening in primary care (Furber AS, *BJGP* 2001;51:757, asymptomatic <25 yo).

Cholesterol trials

- WOSCOPS (prevention of CHD with pravastatin in men with hyper-cholesterolaemia Shepherd J *et al*, *NEJM* 1995;333:1301—TCH >6.5 mmol/L and no h/o CHD on pravastatin for 5 yrs decreased CVD).

- 4S Trial (*Lancet* 1994;344:1383, simvastatin decreases relative risk of coronary mortality in patients with known IHD and TCH 5.5–8 mmol/L).
- CARE 1998 (cholesterol and recurrent events trial showed that lowering average cholesterol with pravastatin after MI reduced cardiac mortality and incidence of MI—Lewis SJ *et al*, *Ann Intern Med* 1998;129:681).
- Heart protection study (*Lancet* 2002;360:7, 40 mg simvastatin od reduced risk of MI, stroke, and revascularisation by ⅓ even in patients with normal or low cholesterol).

Congestive heart failure (past paper topic)

- SOLVD study (studies of left ventricular dysfunction. *NEJM* 1991;325:293—adding enalapril to patients on conventional treatment (class II/III NYHA) improves symptoms, ↓ mortality and ↓ hospital admissions).
- MERIT-HF study, started in 1997 (beta-blocker metoprolol in addition to standard therapy with diuretic, ACEI and digitalis ↓ total mortality and hospitalisation due to heart failure—*Lancet* 1999;353:2001).
- CIBIS II study (*Lancet* 1999;353:9—cardiac insufficiency bisoprolol study).
- Beta-blockers in combination with ACEI in pts with moderate HF—class II and III NYHA ↓ death rate and hospital admission.
- ELITE study (Pitt B *et al*, *Lancet* 1997;349:747—evaluation of Losartan (ATIIR blocker) in the elderly ↓ mortality compared to placebo).
- RALES—randomised aldactone (aldosterone receptor antagonists) evaluation study (Pitt B *et al*, *NEJM* 1999;341:709—only patients with NYHA class III/IV grade of heart failure).
- Spironolactone—one recent large RCT with severe HF found adding aldosterone receptor antag further ↓ mortality.
- Digitalis investigation group (*NEJM* 1997;336:525; effect of digoxin on mortality and morbidity in patients with heart failure—no effect on mortality but ↓ hospital admission in patients with severe HF.

Consent

- Fraser competence, House of Lords.

Diabetes

- UKPDS (UK prospective diabetic study, Turner RC *et al*, *BMJ* 1998;316:823, >5000 with NIDDM over 10 yrs, decrease BP by 10/5 also decreases death from stroke + heart failure; target 140/80).
- HOPE (The Heart Outcomes Prevention Evaluation Study—Yusuf S *et al*, *NEJM* 2000;342:145).
- DIGAMI (DM, insulin glucose infusion in acute MI)—emphasise decrease BP and use of ACEI to decrease CV risk in DM (Malmberg K, *BMJ* 1997;314:1512).

Drug misuse (past paper topic)

- Drug misuse and dependence—guidelines on clinical management (Orange Book, DoH 1999).

Exercise

- Benefits of exercise in health and disease (Fentem PH, *BMJ* 1994;308:1291).

Hypertension

- SHEP—systolic hypertension in elderly program (*JAMA* 1991;265:3255—prevention of stroke by antihypertensive therapy in older patients with isolated systolic hypertension).

Leg ulcers (past paper topic)

- Long healing times and low success rates highlight importance of prevention.
- Elderly deteriorate more; vascular ultrasound for venous ulcers; stop smoking for IC.
- Costs to GP and hospital services; safe use of compression bandaging.

Rheumatoid arthritis (past paper topic)

- Rational use of new and existing disease-modifying agents in RA (Kremer JM, *Ann Intern Med* 2001;134:695; efficacy *vs* placebo in RCT of DMARD—leflunomide, etanercept, infliximab).

- Rheumatoid arthritis (Kassimos D *et al*, *Lancet* 2002;359:352—RCT showed DMARDs efficacy when used together with methotrexate).
- Infante R *et al*, *Geriatrics* 2000;55:30, 35, 39—showed efficacy of Cox-2 inhibitors for relief of signs and symptoms of RA.

Smoking (past paper topic)

- *Smoking Kills*. White paper on tobacco (DoH, Dec 1998).
- Comparison of the smoking behaviours and attitudes of smokers who attribute resp sxs to smoking and those who do not (Walters N *et al*, *BJGP* 2002;52:132—6x ↑ intend to stop smoking if think respiratory sys due to smoking).
- 'Smoking cessation: integration of behavioural and drug therapies' (Mallin R, *Am Fam Physician* 2002;65:1107 —Family physicians take advantage of each contact with smokers. Motivational interviewing techniques move pt from pre-contemplation stage to preparation stage where plans are made for initiation of NRT ± bupropion treatment. Group or individual behavioural counselling can facilitate smoking cessation and improve quitting rates. Combined use of behavioural and drug therapies can dramatically improve patient's chances of quitting smoking.
- NRT yield 1-year cessation rate of 14–18% *vs* 10% with placebo and bupropion 1-yr cessation rate 13% higher (*Prescrire Int* 2001;10:163).
- Use of transdermal nicotine patches over 12 weeks is very cost-effective and doubles the success rate of brief advice at 1 year.
- NICE now approves Zyban (bupropion) on NHS (antidepressant structurally related to amphetamine)—initial 6 mo in Ireland; 12 overdose cases of cardiac arrhythmias and fits (Tracey JA *et al*, *Ir Med J* 2002;95:23 bupropion toxicity.)

Atrial fibrillation (past paper topic)

- 'Stroke and TIA. Prevention and management of cerebrovascular events in primary care (Weinberger J, *Geriatrics* 2002;57:38—TIA with carotid stenosis of >70% should be treated surgically. With carotid stenosis <70%, treat with platelet antiaggregation therapy).
- Comorbidity associated with atrial fib: a general practice-based study (Carroll K *et al*, *BJGP* 2001;51:884, 889—anticoagulation treatment with warfarin ↓ risk of stroke in patients with atrial fib; 40% of patients with atrial fib in primary care are at high risk of stroke and have no C/I for antithrombotic therapy).
- Does the Birmingham model of oral anticoagulation management in primary care work outside trial conditions (Fitzmaurice DA *et al*, *BJGP* 2001;51:828—concludes oral anticoagulation management is safe).

TV0SS14

Thrombolysis

- ISIS-2 benefit of early thrombolysis. Streptokinase ↓ death from MI 25% and ASA further 25%.
- GRAMPIAN—Grampian region early antistreplase trial; 311 patients treated 139 min earlier than within hospital had improved mortality. GP thrombolysis is appropriate.

Terminally ill

- ABC of palliative care: communication with patients, families and other professionals (Faulkner A, *BMJ* 1998;316:130).

Health promotion

- Health promotion in the general practice consultation: a minute makes a difference. Wilson A *et al* (*BMJ* 1992;304:227)—recording of BP, wt, cervical cytology, advice about smoking, alcohol, diet, exercise and immunisation.

British Journal of General Practice Hot Topics, Papers 2001–2002

May 2001   Diagnosis of heart failure in primary care: an assessment of international guidelines

June 2001   Women who experience domestic violence

- Health-care issues, professional need for training

July 2001   *Chlamydia trachomatis*: opportunistic screening in primary care

- Asymptomatic females <25 yo should have had FVU
- Treat with azithromycin 1g or amox for 3 days

Frequent attenders in general practice, retrospective 20-yr follow-up

- Elderly females are 94% with chronic health problems

Meeting the NSF for CHD. Which patients have untreated BP?

- PCT identifies high risk and treat high BP in >65 yo, previously 85% of population's CVD. NSF April 2002, identify patients with 10-year risk of CV >30% and provide advice and treatment to ↓ SBP by 10 mm Hg corresponds to ↓ in 14% of a CV event

Aug 2001   Dyspepsia in primary care: to prescribe or to investigate?

- H2RAs initial treatment for reflux symptoms
- Check *H pylori* status in ulcer-like dyspepsia
- *H pylori*-negative with ulcer-like dyspepsia → short course of PPI
- Nonspecific symptoms—upper endoscopy ± abdominal U/S
  - — (Early endoscopy not for uncomplicated dyspepsia)
  - — If negative, does not require medical attention
  - — 'Wait and see' in young pt
- If predominant symptom is pain, omeprazole is better than H2RA
- Prokinetic treatment (cisapride) for non-specific complaint—fallen into disrepute
- Glasgow study—smoking + obesity RFs are more important than HP

- Danish study—no difference in symptoms 1 year after follow-up with early endoscpy and 44.52 treatment with ranitidine 150 mg bd
- PPI for ulcer-like dyspepsia or uninvestigated dyspepsia

Clinical diagnosis of influenza virus infection: evaluation of diagnostic tools in general practice

- PPV 75% combination of headache, fever, and cough
- PPV for diagnosis by GP judgement is 76%
- Nose throat swab PCR increases detection of viral pathogenesis over viral culture

Sept 2001   Aspirin use for the prevention of CVD

- GPs need to identify individuals with CVD and put on aspirin

Oct 2001   Needs assessment of women with urinary incontinence in a district health authority

Clinical RF as predictor of postmenopausal osteoporosis in general practice

Is population coronary heart disease risk screening justified?

- Discussion of the NSF for CHD

Nov 2001   MMR and the age of unreason

- *Lancet* suggested causal link with IBD and autism
- DoH no good scientific evidence to support link
- Separate vaccines increase risk of children catching disease

Comorbidity associated with atrial fibrillation: a GP-based study

- Annual risk stroke 4–8% with atrial fib: 40% of patients with atrial fib in primary care have increased risk of stroke and no contraindications to antithrombolytic therapy. C/I: congenital defect, psychiatric, dementia, PUD, CA, degenerative disorder, cerebral, PD, epilepsy, GI bleed, chronic hepatitis/cirrhosis, acute or chronic renal failure

Dec 2001   Aetiology of respiratory tract infections: clinical assessment *vs* serological tests

- Doctor's clinical assessment potluck viral *vs* bacterial *vs* atypical

Systematic review of RCT of Viagra in the treatment of erectile dysfunction (effective)

Jan 2002	Patient and career satisfaction with 'Hospital at Home' quantitative and qualitative results from a RCT
	Exercise training and heart failure: a systematic rev of current evidence
Feb 2002	Comparison of smoking behaviour and attitude of smokers who attribute respiratory symptoms to smoking and those who do not
	Cardiovascular RFs and diseases in general practice: results of the Nijmegen Cohort Study
	Predicting the outcome of sciatica at short-term follow-up
March 2002	Antibiotic prescribing and admissions with major suppurative complications of respiratory tract infections: a data linkage study
	Thrombosis prevention trial: follow-up studies of practical implication
	Effect of diabetic control or incidence of, and changes in, retinopathy in Type II NIDDM patients
April 2002	Supporting S Asian carers and those they care for: the role of the PCT

British Journal of General Practice Hot Topics, Papers 2001–2002

RCGP Examination: Instructions and Glossary

THE ROYAL COLLEGE OF GENERAL PRACTITIONERS

EXAMINATION FOR MEMBERSHIP

WRITTEN PAPER ONE

Candidate's Name ....
(BLOCK CAPITALS)

INSTRUCTIONS*

Questions 2, 3, and 12 require you to use additional reference material. The reference material for questions 2 and 3 is taken from the same published paper. You should read the question first, and then the reference material. An extra 30 minutes is allowed for you to read the material for these three questions.

The total time for the paper is therefore 3½ hours.

- Markers do not receive this sheet showing your name, so please check that your number is correct on all pages.
- There are 12 questions in this paper. You may attempt them in any order you wish.
- Each of the 12 questions presented will be marked by a different examiner. It may be necessary therefore for you to repeat parts of an earlier answer or answers if this is relevant to the question you are answering.
- Answers should be legible and concise. You may use 'notes' form.
- Answers should be written in the space provided on the question sheet. You may continue your answer on the reverse of the same sheet. Additional paper may be obtained from the invigilator if necessary.
- References from journals and books should be mentioned if these are relevant to the arguments being presented.

*Reproduced with permission from the RCGP.

Glossary[*]

Comment—write notes to explain, critically.

Example: The data (shown below) come from drug company promotional literature that was being presented to GPs at an educational meeting. *Comment* on the study method.

This requires the candidate both to explain what the study method is as well as to do so critically, by considering its appropriateness for the problem under consideration.

Discuss—consider and debate.

Example: Your new partner asks for help in persuading the other partners to change to longer appointment times. *Discuss* in terms of the new partner and partnership.

A good answer would both consider the views of the new partner and the partnership and debate the value of longer appointments, including some reference to relevant literature.

Implication—something that is suggested or hinted at.

Example: What are the *implications* of revalidation for general practitioners in the United Kingdom?

The question invites the candidate to consider a wide range of issues, including practical, political, ethical and attitudinal ones, suggested by revalidation. Implications in this and other cases might include past, present, and future dimensions of the issue or problem.

Issue—a topic of interest or discussion or one requiring a decision, an important subject.

Example: Cameron Murray has at last got a job on an oil rig subject to a satisfactory 'medical'. The employer requires a routine drug screen. It is reported to you as positive for cannabis. What *issues* does this raise?

In this question there are some more obvious issues, such as the safety of a drug user working on an oil rig, and some less obvious ones—the 'at last' implies that Cameron has been searching for a job for some time.

Manage(ment)—in a medical context management usually includes relevant history taking, examination, treatment, investigation, and referral. In answer to a question explaining management in general practice it may be relevant to address the use of appropriate consultation skills.

Respond—act or react.

Example: Reports from your local hospital have given you serious concerns about nursing standards in the local hospital. How might you *respond*?

A good answer would include a wide range of responses including the gathering of evidence and a number of possible ways in which the identified problems can be addressed.

Process—the method of doing or producing something.

Example: A woman aged 75 has fallen and fractured her hip in a local nursing home.   Discuss a 'significant event analysis' ... in terms of *process*, prevention and outcome.

The process of a significant event analysis in this example would include the ways in which the meeting was introduced, a discussion of who would be invited, and the way in which the meeting was run.

Factor—a contributing element or cause.

Example: Comfort Tetsola, a 45-year-old Afro-Caribbean woman, has a BMI of 45. What *factors* would influence your management?

Relevant elements in this case would include factors relevant to the individual patient (e.g., her motivation to address the problem); to you the doctor (e.g. your skill and knowledge), and other issues, such as medical causes and the availability of resources.

*Reprinted with permission of the RCGP.

Written Paper One

For the Royal College of General Practitioners' Instructions and Glossary for the Written Paper Module, see pages 18–19

Question 1

Farah Shah, aged 40 years, attends for a pap smear. You notice she has multiple bruises on her arms and legs of different ages.

What issues does this raise?

Question 2

Please refer to **Reference material A** (part of an abstract from a paper entitled: Penicillin for acute sore throat in children: randomised, double blind trial) and answer the questions listed below.

a) Comment on the strengths and weaknesses of the methodology of this study.

b) What further information about the methodology would you wish to obtain from the paper in its entirety?

Reference Material A
(Question 2)

Penicillin for acute sore throat in children: randomised, double blind trial.
Zwart S, Rovers MM, de Melker RA, Hoes AW.
BMJ *2003* Dec;327:1324–1326.

Participants and methods

Overall 308 children aged 4–15 contacted their general practitioner because of an acute sore throat. We included children who had a sore throat for less than 7 days and at least two of the four Centor criteria (history of fever, absence of cough, swollen tender anterior cervical lymph nodes, and tonsillar exudate). We excluded severely ill children. Of the 240 eligible children 156 were randomly assigned to one of three treatment groups: penicillin V for 7 days (n=46), penicillin V for 4 days (n=54), or placebo for 7 days (n=56). The dosage was one 250 mg capsule three times daily for children aged 4–10 and two 250 mg capsules three times daily for children aged 10 and older.

The patients were randomly assigned according to a computer generated list that was blinded to both patients and doctors. The figure shows the flow of patients through the trial.

Throat swabs were taken after randomisation, then again after 2 weeks and a diary was given to the parents. During the study they recorded the children's attendance at school and possible side effects of penicillin.

The primary outcome variable was the duration of symptoms, defined as the number of days of symptoms after randomisation until the pain had resolved permanently. Secondary outcome variables included mean consumption of analgesics (in days), absence from school, development of streptococcal sequelae such as an (imminent) quinsy, eradication of the initial pathogen after 2 weeks, and recurrent episodes of sore throat during the 6 month follow-up period.

The trial had 90% power to detect a difference of one day in the duration of symptoms between groups. With at least 52 children in each of the three groups a difference of one-day duration of symptoms could be detected at a 5% level of significance with 90% power. For subgroup analysis a total of 20 children per group would be needed to detect a difference of 1.5 days of duration of symptoms. We performed all analyses on an intention to treat basis.

Question 3

Tables from the results section of the paper referred to in question 2 (Penicillin for acute sore throat in children: randomised, double blind trial) are provided (please refer to **Reference material B**).

a) **Interpret the results in Tables 1–4.**

b) **How might the evidence influence your current practice?**

Reference Material B
(Question 3)

Penicillin for acute sore throat in children: randomised, double blind trial.

Zwart S, Rovers MM, de Melker RA, Hoes AW.

BMJ *2003 Dec;*327:1324–1326.

Reproduced with permission from the BMJ Publishing Group.

Table 1 Mean duration of sore throat (in days, with 95% confidence intervals) in the three treatment groups

Culture	No of patients	Duration of penicillin treatment per group		
		7 days	3 days	Placebo group
All	156	3.8 (3.2–4.4)	4.6 (4.0–5.2)	3.8 (3.3–4.3)
Positive for group A Strep	96	3.0 (2.4–3.6)	4.8 (4.0–5.6)	3.5 (2.9–4.1)
Other or negative	60	4.9 (4.1–5.7)	4.4 (3.6–5.4)	4.7 (3.5–5.9)

Table 2 Mean duration of absence from school in days (with 95% confidence intervals) in the three treatment groups.

Treatment group	Duration of penicillin treatment per group		
	0 days	7 days	3 days
All (n=156)	2.4 (1.8–3.0)	2.3 (1.7–2.9)	2.8 (2.2–3.5)
Children with group A Strep (n=96)	2.2 (1.6–2.8)	2.2 (1.3–3.0)	2.5 (1.8–3.1)
Children without group A Strep (n=60)	3.2 (1.6–4.7)	2.4 (1.6–3.3)	3.3 (2.0–4.6)

Table 3 Episodes of URTI and sore throat reported by parent or carer during the 6-month follow-up period. Values are numbers (percentages) of patients with at least one episode per given period of treatment group.

	Duration of penicillin treatment per group			
	7 days	3 days	0 days	P value (χ^2 test)
URTI:				
Day 8–15	8/39 (20)	8/39 (20)	7/40 (18)	0.9
Day 16–180	32/39 (82)	31/39 (80)	30/40 (75)	0.5
Sore throat:				
Day 8–15	4/39 (10)	6/39 (15)	4/40 (10)	0.8
Day 16–180	24/39 (62)	18/39 (46)	18/40 (45)	0.2
Children with group A Strep (n=96)	2.2 (1.6–2.8)	2.2 (1.3–3.0)	2.5 (1.8–3.1)	
Children without group A Strep (n=60)	3.2 (1.6–4.7)	2.4 (1.6–3.3)	3.3 (2.0–4.6)	

Table 4 Mean consumption of analgesics (in days with 95% confidence intervals) in the three randomised groups.

		Duration of penicillin treatment per group		
Culture	No of patients	7 days	3 days	Placebo group
All	156	1.1 (0.7–1.6)	1.4 (1.0–1.9)	1.4 (1.0–1.8)
Positive for group A Strep	96	0.8 (0.3–1.3)	1.3 (0.7–1.9)	1.2 (0.8–1.6)
Other or negative	60	1.6 (0.7–2.5)	1.6 (0.9–2.3)	2.0 (1.1–2.9)

Question 4

Doris Branch, aged 80 years, arrives 20 minutes late for her routine appointment smelling of urine and faeces.

How would you manage this consultation?

Question 5

Discuss the factors that a practice might consider in deciding whether or not to screen its female patients for chlamydia infection.

Question 6

Discuss patient participation in primary care in the following areas:

a) Patient groups

b) The doctor–patient consultation

c) The practice

d) Local health care

Question 7

Comment on the following, giving evidence to support your views:

a) Treatment of frozen shoulder

Comments	Evidence

b) Treatment of low back pain

Comments	Evidence

c) Treatment of rheumatoid arthritis

Comments	Evidence

Question 8

70-year-old Sarah Rowe says she can no longer cope with her 75-year-old husband, Bill, who is bed-bound after a debilitating stroke.

In what ways can you help?

Question 9

The homeless are a population that GPs come across. **Comment on the following:**

a)   Describe the homeless population.

b)   What is the role of the GP regarding the homeless?

c)   Why do the homeless have trouble accessing care?

d)   What can be done to address the needs of this population?

Question 10

You must inform Mr Arthur Miller, aged 75, that he may have Parkinson's disease.

How would you manage this consultation? Discuss all relevant issues.

Question 11

Discuss the issues surrounding uncertainty for the patient and doctor within the consultation.

a) Define uncertainty and how it affects the consultation.

b) How can a GP manage uncertainty?

Question 12

Please read the extract from the paper entitled: Community pulmonary rehabilitation after hospitalisation for acute exacerbations of chronic pulmonary disease: randomised controlled study (please refer to **Reference material C**), and answer the question given below.

Comment on the strengths and weaknesses of the methodology of this study.

Reference Material C
(Question 12)

Community pulmonary rehabilitation after hospitalisation for acute exacerbations of chronic obstructive pulmonary disease: randomised controlled study.
Man WD, Polkey MI, Donaldson N, Gray BJ, Moxham J.
BMJ *2004 Nov*;329:1209–1210.

Methods

Patients
The authors recruited 42 patients admitted to King's College Hospital in London with a primary diagnosis of acute exacerbation of COPD. Exclusion criteria included comorbidity that could limit exercise training.

All admitted patients received standard treatment, including nebulised bronchodilators, oxygen, oral or intravenous antibiotics, non-invasive ventilation (if required), and a 1–2 week course of oral prednisolone (30–40 mg daily). On discharge from hospital, patients were allocated to either an early pulmonary rehabilitation programme (within 10 days of hospital discharge) or usual care, using the minimisation method.

Assessment
The authors made baseline assessments in the 24 hours before patients were discharged from hospital and assigned to the intervention, and at 3 months. The authors measured exercise capacity by the incremental shuttle walk test, which is reproducible after a single practice walk. The authors used the St George's respiratory questionnaire (SGRQ) and the chronic respiratory questionnaire (CRQ). The authors measured generic health status with the medical outcomes short form 36 item questionnaire (SF-36). Owing to the nature of the intervention and financial and logistic considerations, it was not possible to blind the patients or the assessors.

Pulmonary rehabilitation
A multidisciplinary team ran the pulmonary rehabilitation programme, which consisted of two classes per week for 8 weeks. Each class lasted 2 hours, consisting of 1 hour of exercise (aerobic walking and cycling, strength training for the upper and lower limb) and 1 hour of educational activities (with an emphasis on self-management of the disease, nutrition,

and lifestyle issues). Respiratory physiotherapists and nurses supervised the exercise component, as did health care based fitness instructors.

Physiotherapists, respiratory nurses, an occupational therapist, an advisor, a social worker, a pharmacist, and a lay member of a patients' group supervised education activities on a rolling rota. Patients also received individualised home exercise programmes, which encouraged at least 20 minutes of exercise per day.

Question 1: Answers

Farah Shah, aged 40 years, attends for a pap smear. You notice she has multiple bruises on her arms and legs of different ages.

What issues does this raise?

Domestic violence affects 1 in 4 women.

Issues for the patient

- Fear of social and economic isolation in her culture.
- Financial problems.
- Use of a 'calling card' to reveal her true agenda.
- Sense of helplessness and low self-esteem leading to increased psychiatric morbidity.
- Without intervention the problem may escalate.
- Fear of husband's retribution (cultural issues).
- Separation or divorce may not be a cultural option.
- History of depression?
- Concern for safety of her children.

Communication issues

- Communication difficulties, as patient may have different cultural beliefs from doctor.
- Language barrier. Need for an interpreter?
- Difficulty for the doctor just to ask.
- Doctor needs to stress confidentiality to patient.

Issues for the doctor

- Assess present situation. Ask if her husband has been abusing her. Ask about her source of support, living circumstances.
- Be sensitive. Respect patient's culture, religion, ethnicity.
- Is the husband a patient in the practice? Need to address any issues for him—alcohol, anger management, etc.
- Clear documentation—verbatim history, time, and dates. Description of injuries (photograph?). Conduct psychological and physical exam.

- Cues: evasive manner, history of attempted suicide, depression, unexplained injuries.
- Explain physical and emotional consequences of ongoing abuse.
- Explain domestic violence is illegal and the patient is a victim.
- Self-awareness—lack of confidence in ability to help.
- Arrange follow-up.

Legal and ethical issues

- Provide written information on legal options and help from police domestic violence units.
- Inform her of the Women's Aid National Helpline and local shelter.
- Are children in danger? Assess need to notify local authorities, social services, child protection team, health visitors.

Practice issues

- Screening for domestic violence in women.

Evidence-based medicine

- Could health professionals screen women for domestic violence? Systematic review. *BMJ*;324:314–318. 50–75% of women found screening acceptable.

Question 2: Answers

Please read the extract from the paper entitled 'Penicillin for acute sore throat in children: randomised, double blind trial (please refer to **Reference material A**) and answer the questions given below.

a)   **Comment on the strengths and weaknesses of the methodology of this study.**

Strengths

Design
- Good randomised double-blinded prospective trial which was placebo controlled.
- Repeatable.
- Instruments—throat swabs (reliable and valid in general practice) but diary (not so good as too subjective).

Subjects
- Good age range of 4–15 years.
- Good initial sample size of 308 children.
- Use of controls.
- Selection was without bias.
- Power was calculated.
- Confidence intervals were included.
- Sample size changed slightly—losing 17 of 156 to follow-up is not bad.
- Experiment is reproducible.
- Treatment plan is clear.
- Time span was defined.

Setting
- GP relevant.

Outcome measures
- Double blinded to patient and clinician by a computer-generated list.
- Relevant outcomes are included in the graph.

Weaknesses

Design
- Confounding variables—severely ill were excluded.
- Treatment is not valid—should be penicillin qds and not tds.
- Instrument (diary) was recorded by parents and not the children, so not reliable.
- p value was not <0.05 in Table 3 so could be due to chance.

Subjects
- 152 of the 308 children were excluded—very high and may bias results.

Setting
- Netherlands and not UK (foreign-based study)

b) **What further information about the methodology would you wish to obtain from the paper in its entirety?**

Design

- Is there a gold standard for comparison?

Subjects

- What is the socioeconomic class of children and families? May have different literacy levels if the instrument is parents keeping a diary.
- What are the defining criteria for the severely ill children who were excluded; as almost a third of the numbers of children were excluded (of 308 children only 156 were eligible), this will influence the results.

Intervention

- Type and amount of analgesia given to subjects may have influenced the outcome.
- What was the placebo?

Outcome measures

- As the initial number of children was 308 and only 156 were selected for the randomised trial, the outcome variables may be biased.

Question 3: Answers

Tables from the results section of the paper referred to in question 2 (Penicillin for acute sore throat in children: randomised, double blind trial) are provided (please refer to **Reference material B**).

a) **Interpret the results in Tables 1–4.**

Table 1

- Suggests that the duration of sore throat in children who test positive for group A strep is not influenced by whether they receive penicillin or not. It suggests that taking penicillin for 7 days shortens the duration of sore throat by 1.8 days as compared to treatment for 3 days. However, it also suggests that no penicillin (i.e., in the placebo group) shortens duration of sore throat by 1.3 days as compared to treatment with penicillin for 3 days!

Table 2

- Suggests that the mean duration of absence from school in days is not affected by whether the child is treated with penicillin or not.

Table 3

- Suggests that the number of episodes of URTI and sore throat during the 6-month follow-up period is not influenced by whether the child was initially treated with penicillin or not.
- However, as the p value is not <0.05, the results may have been due to chance and may not be valid.

Table 4

- Suggests that the mean consumption of analgesics is not influenced by whether the child has received penicillin treatment or not.
- I would like to have seen whether each group were offered the same analgesic and what type of analgesic was offered as this may have biased the results.

Overall I am concerned that 45 children were excluded for being 'severely ill' as their omission has biased the results. This study suggests that penicillin treatment for positive group A strep sore throat may not be necessary!

b) **How might the evidence influence your current practice?**

- I would be sceptical of this study as there are omissions and bias is introduced as of the initial 308 eligible children 152 were excluded for medical reasons and only 156 were eventually used in the study.
- My current mode of practice is to offer penicillin to children who either test positive for group A strep or who are severely ill (unable to drink, quinsy, trismus, peritonsillar cellulitis, etc).
- In conclusion, I would not change my current practice from reading this paper.

Question 4: Answers

Doris Branch, aged 80 years, arrives 20 minutes late for her routine appointment smelling of urine and faeces.

How would you manage this consultation?

Issues for the patient

- Assess mental status—dementia, depression, alcohol misuse.
- Social issues—social isolation, ability to take care of self, home situation, lives alone?
- Embarrassment—incontinence?, stigma attached to problem.
- Hidden issues—abuse by carer?, stress, low self-esteem?
- Loss of autonomy.
- Low expectations of GP management of urinary incontinence—inevitable with age. Regular faecal incontinence or one-off?

Issues for the doctor

- Assess physical, psychological, and social situation. Appropriate history and physical exam to exclude medical cause for urinary and faecal incontinence.
- Acknowledge resentment at tardiness of patient and pressures of time constraints. Accept need to catch-up later during the clinic session so that you are more relaxed when seeing this patient instead of feeling rushed and stressed.
- Communication—use layman's terms, establish rapport, deal with sensitive topic, explore her understanding of incontinence.
- Non-judgmental but acknowledge personal attitude to smelly patients.
- Perform medical assessment to exclude stress incontinence, urge incontinence, UTI, post-micturition dribble, unpredictable leaking without obvious reason with abdominal, PV exam, and MSU, and causes of faecal incontinence with PR exam.
- Respect self-esteem of Doris.
- Offer sympathy.
- Opportunistic health promotion.
- Shared care/referral to community incontinence nurse/CMHT.
- Involvement of social worker, follow-up.
- Need for female chaperone present to examine for urethral prolapse, PV and PR exam.

Practice issues/wider issues/ethics

- Policy on late arrivals—20 minutes? Reschedule? Cancel?
- Encourage more females with incontinence to see GP—posters in waiting room, toilets.
- Improve public, patient, and professional awareness.
- Guidelines of PCT.

Support and follow-up

- Will need annual elderly review of home and person.

Evidence

- Mackay K *et al*, *BJGP* 2001;51:801. Needs assessment of women with urinary incontinence in a district health authority. Only a quarter of women with urinary incontinence consult their doctor despite evidence of effective treatments and better management of the condition in primary care. Cross-sectional community survey ≥45 yo, 68% questionnaires returned (489/720). Of the 46% (227) of the women with significant urinary incontinence, 16% (78) said it was not a problem, 30% (149) said it was a problem, and 32% (48) saw their GP. Of this 32%, 32 were not happy with the GP's management and 16 were happy. The reasons women gave for not seeing their GP were that they could cope on their own (43%) or believed incontinence was inevitable with age (26%).
- Stoddart H, *BJGP* 2001;51:548. Urinary incontinence in older people in the community: a neglected problem? Bristol cross-sectional survey of 11 general practices—2000 patients between 65 and 74 yo, both sexes. Only 40% male and 45% females accessed health services.

Question 5: Answers

Discuss the factors that a practice might consider in deciding whether or not to screen its female patients for chlamydia infection.

Why?

Chlamydia has been recognised by the Chief Medical Officer's Expert Advisory Group as a condition that requires a detailed preventative strategy. It is the most common STD (89,500 cases in 2003) and costs the NHS >£100 million a year. In June 2004, a Health Protection Agency study concluded that there were marked differences in GP knowledge of chlamydia and in the testing rates of practices. The consequences of untreated chlamydia include PID, infertility, and chronic pelvic pain. It is therefore an important condition and worthy of screening, particularly in those at risk.

Implications?

- Cost implications for the practice.
- Time and resource implications—extra staffing, extra sessions?
- Ethical issues—chlamydia screening offered to female patients at one general practice presents as inequality of provision of services and female patients at other practices may make demands to be provided with this service too.
- Ethical issues—maintaining patient confidentiality and obtaining consent for patient participation in screening programme.
- Selection process—all registered female patients? Not cost-effective.
- Ideal target population: all symptomatic females, those seeking TOP, females under 25 screened opportunistically, and those over 25 who have had a recent change in partner.

How?

- Decide on screening tool using evidence-based medicine and current guidelines.
- May use Wilson and Jungner 'IATROGENIC' for screening criteria:
  - *Important* condition—yes; it is the most common STD with implications.

- — *Acceptable* treatment for the disease—yes, with doxycycline 100 mg bd for 1/52 or 1 g of azithromycin stat. For pregnant patients, offer amoxycillin 250 mg or azithromycin.
- — *Treatment* and adequate diagnostic facilities available—yes, in GP surgery or local GUM clinics.
- — *Recognisable* latent or early symptomatic stage—yes, but can be asymptomatic.
- — *Opinions* on who to treat are agreed—will need to agree in practice meeting.
- — *Guaranteed* safety and reliability of test (see testing below).
- — *Examination* acceptable to patient—urine test is less invasive than endocervical swabs.
- — *Natural history of disease* is known—yes.
- — *Inexpensive* and simple test suitable—yes.
- — *Continuous*—repeated at intervals determined by natural history of disease.
- — Testing. This is based on nucleic acid amplification such as ligase (polymerase) chain reaction analysis, which can be performed on a first-void urine sample or virology on endocervical swabs.
- — Treatment. Treatment is as mentioned above with doxycycline or azithromycin, condoms advised for SI, and attendance at GUM clinic also advised for aftercare, partner notification, and further STD testing.

Evidence-based medicine

- Tobin C *et al*, *BJGP* 2001;51:565, Chlamydia trachomatis: opportunistic screening in primary care. 10.9% prevalence in GP surgery in West Yorkshire. CMO—screen asymptomatic sexually-active females under 25. Use of FVU (first void urine) posters in waiting rooms. Sample is frozen overnight at −22 °C or refrigerate at 2 °C and transport to lab for polymerase chain reaction analysis.

Question 6: Answers

Discuss patient participation in primary care in the following areas:

a) **Patient groups**

Public expectations are rising faster than the ability of health services to meet them.
- Recognise patient's expertise, values and preferences.
- Offer informed choice and not passive consent.
- Offer training in shared decision making. Time consuming and expensive.
- Provide evidence-based decision aids for patients.
- Provide public education on interpreting clinical evidence.
- Confidentiality issue arises if patients have access to electronic health records.
- Offer survey of patients' experience to prioritise quality improvements.
- Openness and empathy with patients after medical errors have occurred.
- Issue of public access to comparative data on quality and outcomes.
- However elderly still like the paternalistic approach.
- How to get patients from all sectors (all stakeholders) involved? Postal/telephone poll? Some patients may have personal agenda and may not be representative. May be more educated and more vocal with their own health agenda. How to target the homeless, illiterate, vulnerable, etc?
- Evidence-based medicine: Coulter A, *BMJ* 2002;324:648. After Bristol: Putting patients at the centre by Angela Coulter

b) **The doctor–patient consultation**

- Involve the patient (or parents) in decision-making process.
- Elicit feedback from patients.
- Effect of increased time constraints on allowing time for an empathetic approach.
- Give informed consent for all processes and procedures, adverse outcomes.
- Appropriateness and outcome of care can be improved by engaging patients in treatment and management decisions.
- Elicit patient's beliefs and preferences about medicine to minimise poor compliance.
- Quality of clinical communication—use layman's terms.
- Patient-centred consultation may not suit all GPs—consumer based.

c) **The practice**

- Regular, systematic feedback from patients is essential to improve quality of care and for public accountability.

- Physical access to all patients to include location of building and its layout.
- Timing and availability of appointments.
- Systems of communication in place.
- Needs assessment on a local and national/statutory basis to confirm compliance with standards.
- Changes and primary health-care team—resistance and enthusiasm.
- Limited resources (financial implications) so patient group needs may not all be met. Allocation of services.

d) **Local health care**

- Survival of the NHS depends on the extent to which it can respond to patients' needs and wishes.
- Safety can be improved and complaints and litigation reduced if patients are actively involved in their own care.
- Budgetary pressures from government.
- Publication of performance indicators that allow health-care facilities to be compared.
- There is more lay representation in the PCTs, GMC, and RCGP. Is it appropriate for a lay representative to assess a GP's fitness to practise without appropriate medical training? How much involvement by patients is too much?

Question 7: Answers

Comment on the following, giving evidence to support your views:

a) **Treatment of frozen shoulder**

Comments	Evidence
Criteria at least 1/12 + PE painful restricted shoulder motion but most recover with or without treatment within 2 years from onset	
Algorithm 90% good results with gentle home programme of passive stretching	Goldberg BA et al, J Orthop Sci 1999;4:462 Dept of Ortho, Univ of Wash. Management of stiff shoulder
↓	
MUA	
↓	
Arthroscopic release of capsular contractures + aggressive rehab programme	Pearsall AW, et al, Med Sci Sports Exerc 1988;30:533
NSAIDs + oral corticosteroids	Dept of Ortho Surgery Frozen shoulder syndrome: Diagnostic and treatment strategies in the primary care setting
Surgical intervention if MUA not effective	
Intra-articular steroid injections	
Bupivacaine suprascapular nerve blocks effective in decreasing pain of frozen shoulder at 1 month	Dahan TH et al, J Rheumatol 2000;27:1464 Double-blinded RCT examining the efficacy of bupivacaine supra-scapular nerve blocks in frozen shoulder
Manipulation under GA	Dodenhoff RM, J Shoulder Elbow Surg 2000;9:23 MUA for primary frozen shoulder. Effective for early recovery and return to activity

Comments	Evidence
1. Corticosteroids	*BJGP* 2002 Feb 94% definitive evidence short-term efficacy
2. NSAIDs	89% of clinicians and systematic critical review for short-term efficacy
3. Movement exercise or mobilisation	No evidence for efficacy
4. Acupuncture	Tentative evidence
5. Ultrasound therapy and TENS	Tentative evidence for lack of efficacy
6. Strengthening exercise—physio	Better outcome than no treatment

b) **Treatment of low back pain**

Comments	Evidence
Outlines criteria to exclude serious spinal pathology, red flags	*Clinical Guidelines for the Management of Acute LBP* RCGP, Waddell G *et al, BJGP* 1997;47:647
Analgesia at regular intervals	Management of acute LBP, DTB 1998
No evidence that coproxamol or codydramol is superior to paracetamol alone Short-term use of muscle relaxants better than placebo Early return to normal physical activity leads to more rapid recovery Bedrest is not advised Muscles lose 3% of their strength per day Refer for physio if no better after 6/52 90% recover within 6 weeks	RCGP. Management of acute LBP, 1999 *Clinical Evidence*, June 2004

c) **Drug treatment of rheumatoid arthritis**

Comments	Evidence
NSAIDs traditional + methotrexate + cyclosporine	*Lancet* 2002 Jan Rheumatoid arthritis RCT and observational studies showed increased efficacy and acceptable toxicity

Comments	Evidence
Selective Cox-2 inhibitors	*Geriatrics* 2000 Mar Efficacy similar to NSAIDs but with less GI and platelet toxicity
Old disease-modifying anti-rheumatic drugs (hydroxycholoroquine, sulfasalazine)	Kremer JM, *Ann Intern Med* 2001;134:615 Rational use of new and existing disease-modifying agents in RA
New DMARDs TNF antagonists (leflunomide, etanercept, infliximab) Infliximab—monoclonal mouse antibody against TNF-alpha	Slows disease activity and progression USA approved in 1999 NICE approved for infliximab and etanercept for treatment of RA
Etanercept + methotrexate	TEMPO study showed that combination was better than methotrexate alone
Infliximab + methotrexate	ATTRACT trial showed infliximab + methotrexate retards radiographic progress versus methotrexate alone

Question 8: Answers

70-year-old Sarah Rowe says she can no longer cope with her 75-year-old husband, Bill, who is bed-bound after a debilitating stroke.

In what ways can you help?

There are 6 million informal carers in the UK for the aged and disabled or 1 in 7 of the population are carers.

GP's role to support the carer

- Assess coping and offer support, e.g. support groups, respite care.
- Assess need for a break. Carers prone to health problems as a result of their role, stress-related illness, increase in physical injuries, increase in all-cause mortality.
- Look for signs of depression or isolation.
- Open discussion of prognosis.
- Assess need for advice and help.
- Is appropriate help available?

GP's role to provide access to rehabilitation services within PCT for husband

- Assess need for disability aids, access community nursing, home-care services, speech therapy, bathing assistance.
- Arrange occupational therapy assessment and physiotherapy to decrease disability.
- Hospital At Home schemes are on the rise in the UK.
- Local charities.

GP's role in follow-up

- Ongoing need for information, e.g. Stroke Association.
- Consider patient's changing needs and environment.
- Medical review of patient and carer.
- Look for signs of depression in patient and carer.
- Possibility of long-term residential care.

Issues for the GP

- Lack relevant resources and training to take more proactive role.
- See themselves in a reactive role only. Suggest training or access literature.
- Shift from hospital- to community-based care puts added pressure on the carer.
- Supply information about local resources..

Evidence-based medicine

- Simon C et al, BJGP 2001;51:655. Informal carers—the role of GPs and district nurses. Postal survey of 300 GPs and 272 DNs to determine views on role in supporting carers.
- HM Govt. A National Strategy for Carers. London: The Stationery Office, 1999.
- Wilson A et al, BJGP 2002;52:9. Patient and carer satisfaction with 'hospital at home': quantitative and qualitative results from a randomised controlled trial. Conclusion: Patient satisfaction greater with hospital at home—more personal style of care and feeling that staying at home was therapeutic. Carers did not feel that hospital at home was an extra workload.
- Simon C, BJGP 2001;51:920. Informal carers and the primary care team. Suggests:
  - Acknowledge carers, what they do, and the problems they have.
  - Flag notes of informal carers so that in any consultation you are aware of their circumstances.
  - Treat carers as you would other team members and listen to their opinions.
  - Include them in discussions about the person they care for.
  - Give carers a choice about which tasks they are prepared to take on themselves.
  - Ask after the health and welfare of the carer and the patient.
  - Provide information about the condition the patient has.
  - Provide information about being a carer and support available.
  - Provide information about benefits available.
  - Provide information about local services available for both person being cared for and carer.
  - Be an advocate to the carer to ensure services and equipment appropriate to the circumstances are provided.
  - Liaise with other services.
  - Ensure staff are informed about needs and problems of informal carers.
  - Respond quickly and sympathetically to crisis situations.
- Katbama S et al, BJGP 2002;52:300. Supporting S Asian carers and those they care for: the role of the PHCT. DoH National Strategy for Carers.

Question 9: Answers

The homeless are a population that GPs encounter. **Comment on the following:**

a) **Describe the homeless population.**

The homeless or indigent population comprises the following groups:
- Chronic alcohol misusers.
- IV drug misusers.
- Refugees.
- Mental illness sufferers—schizophrenia.
- Dual diagnosis patients.
- Impoverished elderly.
- Impoverished families.
- Victims of domestic violence.

b) **What is the role of the GP regarding the homeless?**

Alcohol and IV drug misusers

According to *Drug Misuse and Dependence—Guidelines on Clinical Management*, Department of Health Orange Book 1999, the role of the GP is as follows:
- Presentation: pregnant, impending court case, wanting help, etc. Confirm patient is taking drugs (history, exam, and urine toxicology screen) or assess degree of alcohol dependence.
- Past and current drug use: age at starting, types, quantity, frequency, and routes of administration, overdoses, abstinences, symptoms (hallucinations, fits). Assess degree of dependence (smoking, injecting, amount per week).
- Medical history—abscess, DVT, chest infections, dental disease, TB, bacterial endocarditis, PE, LMP, last smear, accidents, delirium tremens, seizures, liver disease.
- Psychiatric history—admissions, OPC, overdoses, depression or concomitant psychosis (delusions or hallucinations), self-harm, attempted suicide.
- Forensic history—probation, criminal record, outstanding charges.
- Social history—family, children, employment, accommodation (hostel), debt. Provide long-term medical certificates for mental instability, drug dependence, etc.
- Past contact with treatment services—prior attempts at rehab, methadone, etc. Refer to treatment services.

- Others—alcohol or drug misuse in partner or family. Risk to family members of violence?
- Examine sites of injection for infection (neck, arms, groin, and legs).
- Reduce risk of HIV, hepatitis B and C, and other blood-borne infections from injecting. Offer hepatitis vaccinations.
- Reduce need for criminal activity.
- Reduce use of illicit drugs by the individual.
- Assist patient to remain healthy and stabilise patient on substitute medication.
- Identify complications of drug misuse and assess risk behaviour (skin abscesses, h/o DVT) or complications of alcohol misuse.
- Identify medical, social, and mental health problems.
- Offer advice on harm minimisation (clean needle exchange centres, testing for HIV, and immunisation against hepatitis B).
- Determine patient's expectations and degree of motivation.
- Determine need for substitute medication such as methadone or subutex.
- Notify the patient to the local Regional Drug Misuse Database (form completion).
- Assess the appropriate level of expertise needed for this patient (shared care). Shared care with specialist GPs, community psychiatric nurses, clinical psychologists, pharmacist, social worker, and drug and alcohol workers.
- Refer for specialist services for patients with dual diagnoses (mental illness + drug/alcohol), liver disease, chaotic lifestyle, serious forensic history, unresponsive to oral substitute prescriptions, specialised residential rehabilitation programmes.
- Arrange investigations: Hb, creatinine, LFTs, hepatitis B and C, HIV antibody.
- Urine toxicology test (opiates persist for 24 h and methadone for 48 h).

Refugees

- Provide medical and psychosocial support.
- Refer to refugee council or other support centres.

Mental illness patients

- Involve social worker, refer to CPN, CMT.
- Provide repeat prescriptions.
- Offer psychosocial support .
- Tend to medical needs.
- Familiar with Mental Health Act and aware when to use.
- Offer long-term medical certificates for mental instability.

Impoverished patients

- Refer to social services.
- Offer psychosocial support and address medical needs.

Victims of domestic violence

- Refer to women's national helpline, local authorities social services and housing departments.
- Document injuries and address medical needs.

c) **Why do the homeless have trouble accessing care?**

- Transient lifestyle leads to discontinuity of GP care. Lack of education may impede patients from acquiring care due to lack of knowledge and means to access. May even be illiterate.
- Stigma, shame, prejudice, and embarrassment surrounding homelessness. Being an alcohol or drug misuser may prevent patients from accessing care. These patients regard themselves as on the fringes of society and may be afraid to access 'the establishment.'
- Temporary accommodation in hostels may lead to loss to follow-up upon referral to OPCs, CMT, etc. No permanent postal address or telephone number.
- Language barrier may prevent refugees from accessing care or registering with a local general practice.
- Mental illness may prevent a patient from seeking help when necessary.
- Fear of being reported to the police for illegal activity or illegal status may impede access.

d) **What can be done to address the needs of this population?**

- Encourage more GPs to opt-in to provide services to the homeless, refugees, drug misusers.
- Increase GP awareness with education and local involvement.
- GPs should be more sensitive when addressing a homeless person and allow the person to have dignity and to speak freely, to empower the patient.
- Shelters and hostels should encourage local general practices to get involved.
- More GPs could volunteer to provide on-site medical care at local shelters.
- Encourage politicians and local government to provide more funding to address this population.
- Multidisciplinary approach—local shelters, local GPs, local voluntary organisations, local MPs, national policies, etc.

Evidence

- Lester H *et al*, *BJGP* 2002;52:91. Developments in the provision of primary health care for homeless people.

Question 10: Answers

You must inform Mr Arthur Miller, aged 75, that he may have Parkinson's disease.

How would you manage this consultation? Discuss all relevant issues.

The Government white paper *Saving Lives: Our Healthier Nation* states that one in three people in this country lives with a chronic disease like PD. This has both economical and personal implications for the patient and the health-care services as the population lives longer.

Communication

- Establish a rapport with Arthur Miller.
- Inform him of the suspected diagnosis with caritas and use layman's terms.
- Offer valid information and good communication.
- Use the principles of breaking bad news.
- Need to identify disease early and provide patient with supportive information to ensure positive outlook on the diagnosis and to allow the patient to develop a long-term plan of management.
- Ascertain his understanding of PD and its management.
- Explore his ideas regarding the condition, concerns, and anxieties, and his expectations from you, and try to meet his needs.
- Give him time to reflect and involve family members/potential carers.
- Allow him the opportunity to ask you questions.
- Make use of the Parkinson's Disease Society (PDS) to help communicate the diagnosis. It uses a structured approach involving several consultations with a specialist and employs a multidisciplinary support, involving the patient, key worker, and Parkinson's Disease Nurse Specialist.

Issues for the patient

- Loss of autonomy.
- Fear.
- Depression.
- Feelings of devastation.
- Social support.
- Beliefs with respect to this condition.

Issues for the GP

- Suspect PD if patient presents with a tremor.
- Biomedical model—patient will need to be referred to secondary care to confirm the diagnosis and initiate treatment.
- Self-awareness—uncertainty regarding diagnosis. The differential includes essential tremor, drug-induced parkinsonism (chlorpromazine, haloperidol or metoclopramide), vascular parkinsonism, multisystem atrophy, progressive supranuclear palsy, co-morbidities, etc. Take a good history and examination. Early referral is important as the misdiagnosis rate is high even among neurologists.
- As the diagnosis is a clinical one, use of DatSCAN using FP-CIT available at DGHs or PET scan at specialist centres can aid in confirmation of diagnosis. Again early referral to specialist centres is crucial.
- Self-awareness—feelings of ignorance regarding the condition. Address educational needs—PUNS/DENS.
- Prescribing should be left to specialist services—guidelines suggest initiating therapy with a direct dopaminergic agonist (cabergoline, pergolide, pramipexole, ropinirole), especially in younger patients, before offering therapy with levodopa, to avoid potential motor fluctuations and dyskinesia with high doses. However, dopaminergic agonists are associated with increased treatment withdrawal and poorer motor scores (*Clinical Evidence*). RCTs show that selegiline (MAO B inhibitor) improves the symptoms of mild-to-moderate PD and delays the need for levodopa. RCTs also show that dopamine agonists + levodopa reduce dyskinesia but increase disability.
- Need to discuss and educate patient as to the benefits and side-effects of therapy. Need to inform patient that the tremor does not respond well to standard doses of medication but that bradykinesia responds better. Catechyl-O-methyl transferase (COMT) inhibitors (entacapone) may need to be prescribed with levodopa to alleviate potential side-effects.
- Need to meet health needs of both patient and potential carers, as this is a chronic disabling disease.

Support and follow-up

- Empowering patient—offer continued support and current information to allow patient to assume control.
- Social assessment.
- Offer follow-up for family and patient to address questions that may arise later.
- Refer patient to PDS or GP with specialist interest in neurology as diagnosis and management require a multidisciplinary team.

Wider issues

- Advance directives (living will),
- NSF for the elderly.
- Confidentiality—does he give permission to inform his family?
- Autonomy—respect his rights.
- Implications for society—cost issue of management of chronic disease in a climate of limited existing health-care resources.
- Research needs—PDS supports the development of commissioned specialist research with funding and fellowship programmes. Involvement and funding by local and national charities and by drug companies.

Evidence

- Parkinson Study Group. Dopamine transporter brain imaging to assess the effects of pramipexole vs levodopa on Parkinson disease progression. *JAMA* 2002;287:1653–1661.
- Bhatia KP, Brooks DJ, Burn DJ, *et al.* Updated guidelines for the management of Parkinson's Disease. *Hosp Med* 2001;62:456–470.
- Rascol O, Brooks DJ, Korczyn AD, *et al.* A five-year study of the incidence of dyskinesia in patients with early Parkinson's disease who were treated with ropinirole or levodopa. *NEJM* 2000 May;342:1484–1491.

Question 11: Answers

Discuss the issues surrounding uncertainty for the patient and doctor within the consultation.

a) **Define uncertainty and how it affects the consultation.**

Uncertainty within the consultation covers many areas of uncertainty: uncertainty with respect to the patient's diagnosis and management, patient's hidden agenda, doctor's knowledge base, trust between patient and doctor.

Issues for the doctor

- Doctor may feel inadequate and uncertain as to patient's true diagnosis, best way to treat or manage a condition, or which guideline is applicable. Does the doctor go by clinical experience or use the latest NICE guideline or evidence-based medicine?
- This then becomes a source of stress for the doctor and can lead to burnout if he/she is burdened with too much uncertainty in consultations.
- On a positive note, uncertainty makes the doctor aware of his/her learning needs (PUNS/DENS) and encourages the doctor to educate him/herself.
- Uncertainty imparts to the doctor a duty of responsibility of care and encourages him/her to safety net (ask for advice, arrange follow-up, discuss in practice meeting, liaise with secondary services, use multidisciplinary team approach, etc), if he/she is not 100% happy with the diagnosis or management.
- Doctor may feel burdened by public pressure and ever increasing litigation, and as a result practise defensive medicine to deal with his/her uncertainty. This has expensive cost implications on the health service and prevents the doctor from exercising his/her role as gatekeeper in rationing health care.

Issues for the patient

- Patient may be uncertain as to whether he/she can trust the doctor due to prejudice or past experience.
- Patient may be uncertain as to whether the doctor has made the correct diagnosis and is offering the best management. Patient may doubt doctor's competence.

- Uncertainty in patient's mind has a detrimental effect on the consultation and impedes the patient–doctor relationship/trust, which can then impact negatively on patient compliance with advice, treatment, and follow-up.

b) **How can a GP manage uncertainty?**

- Improve his/her communication skills (both verbal and nonverbal) if he/she senses that the patient is not happy with the consultation.
- Ask for help—from the community, hospital, colleagues, etc.
- Meet his/her educational needs by attending courses, reading, etc.
- Share management options with the patient to encourage patient empowerment and compliance.
- Share with the patient his/her lack of expertise in a particular area and at the same time explain who he/she will contact for advice or to whom he/she will refer the patient, thereby being honest with the patient and building trust and confidence in the patient–doctor relationship.

Question 12: Answers

Please read the extract from the paper entitled: Community pulmonary rehabilitation after hospitalisation for acute exacerbations of chronic pulmonary disease: randomised controlled study (please refer to **Reference material C**) and answer the question given below.

Comment on the strengths and weaknesses of the methodology of this study.

Strengths

- Randomised controlled study with use of controls.
- Study design is repeatable.
- Questionnaires seem reliable and valid.
- Inclusion criteria stated.
- Exclusion criteria defined—comorbidity that could limit training.
- Treatment plan is clearly stated for the intervention group.
- Time span stated.

Weaknesses

- No mention of whether patients are similar in age, sex, ethnicity, and socioeconomic class to avoid confounding variables.
- No clarification of what the 'minimisation method' is for the control group.
- Not blind to the patients or assessors.
- No mention of whether the sample size had changed.
- Power has not been calculated.
- Sample size of 42 patients may not be sufficient to detect statistically significant results.

Written Paper Two

For the Royal College of General Practitioners' Instructions and Glossary for the Written Paper Module, see pages 18–19

Question 1

Your practice is planning a policy on prescribing antidepressants for depression.

Outline how you would gather your evidence.

Question 2

Your practice wishes to develop an evidence-based approach to the treatment of earwax.

a) **How would you ensure a comprehensive inclusion of studies?**

One study that you discover is: The effectiveness of topical preparations for the treatment of earwax: a systematic review.

b) **The authors searched Medline. What are the strengths and weaknesses of Medline as a database?**

Strengths	Weaknesses

Please refer to **Reference material A.**

c) **Discuss the approach adopted by the authors to assess the evidence.**

Reference Material A
(Question 2)

The effectiveness of topical preparations for the treatment of earwax: a systematic review.
Hand C, Harvey I.
BJGP 2004 Nov;54:862–867.

Reproduced with permission from the *BJGP*.

Methods

Two reviewers (CH and IH) examined Medline, CINAHL, and the Cochrane Controlled Trials Register (last accessed January 2004) using the search terms 'ears and wax', 'earwax', 'cerumen', and 'trial'. The reviewers searched the National Research Register (June 2003) for ongoing studies and accessed Clinical Evidence (June 2003) for the most recent advice and references. The reviewers scrutinised the references of the identified articles and also those of many review articles on the management of earwax and ear care. The reviewers contacted experts in the field, people currently doing research on earwax, some of the authors of the identified trials, the pharmaceutical companies manufacturing the preparations used in the UK, and two companies in the US.

The authors included all randomised trials that evaluated drops used for treatment of earwax with no restriction on either date or language. Each trial was read independently to assess its eligibility and quality. The authors excluded non-randomised studies and assessed the quality of the RCTs using the following criteria:

- reported generation of allocation sequence
- allocation concealment
- inclusion of randomised patients, and
- blinding of outcome assessors.

The authors used a three-point scale for each criterion and defined a high-quality trial as having the maximum score on each of the four criteria. The very few differences in opinion were settled by negotiation.

The authors classified eardrops into three groups: water-based, oil-based, and non-water-, non-oil-based. The classification is based on the physical and chemical properties of the preparations, as the mechanisms of action are probably different. The underlying assumption of the classification is that preparations with similar properties have similar mechanisms of action. There is evidence for this from in vitro studies:

water-based preparations have a cerumenolytic activity, whereas oil-based preparations have only a softening effect. There have been no published *in vitro* studies using non-water-, non-oil-based preparations.

When urea-hydrogen peroxide (carbamide peroxide, Exterol), Otex comes into contact with water, hydrogen peroxide is one of the main products. This has been shown to have powerful cerumenolytic activity in vitro. In the 1940s, both hydrogen peroxide (which breaks down into water) and water were shown to have cerumenolytic activity. Cerumenolytics work by hydrating the desquamated sheets of corneocytes, which are the major constituents of cerumen plugs, and subsequently inducing keratolysis with disintegration of the wax.

The main outcomes assessed were clearing earwax without syringing and successful syringing. Successful syringing was variably defined in studies, but included ease of syringing, clearance of wax, and the ability to see the tympanic membrane afterwards. Using a random effects model, the authors pooled the results of studies that compared water-based, oil-based, and non-water-, non-oil-based preparations where the authors could identify suitably similar outcomes, and when the authors were satisfied that the randomisation procedures were acceptable.

Question 3

Tables from the results section of the paper referred to in question 2 (The effectiveness of topical preparations for the treatment of earwax: a systematic review) are provided (please refer to **Reference material B**).

a) **Interpret the results in Tables 2 and 3.**

b) **How might the evidence from Tables 2 and 3 influence your current practice?**

Reference Material B (Question 3)

The effectiveness of topical preparations for the treatment of earwax: a systematic review.
Hand C, Harvey I.
BJGP 2004 Nov;54:862–867.

Reproduced with permission from the *BJGP*.

Table 2 Effectiveness of preparations in clearing earwax.

Study	Docusate (water-based)	TEP (water-based)	Odds ratio (95% CI)
Singer *et al*	5/27	2/23	2.4 (0.3–27.2)
Meehan *et al*	2/15	7/17	0.2 (0.02–1.6)
Whatley *et al*	4/34	4/30	0.9 (0.1–5.2)
Total	11/76	13/70	0.8 (0.2–2.8)
Heterogeneity	Woolf Q = 3.6, df = 2, P = 0.2		
Overall effect	χ^2 = 0.1, df = 1, P = 0.7		
	Docusate (water-based)	**Saline (water-based)**	
Meehan *et al*	2/15	2/16	1.1 (0.07–16.9)
Whatley *et al*	4/34	1/28	3.6 (0.3–183.7)
Total	6/49	3/44	1.9 (0.4–8.8)
Heterogeneity	Woolf Q = 0.6, df = 1, P = 0.4		
Overall effect	χ^2 = 0.7, df = 1, P = 0.4		
	TEP (water-based)	**Saline (water-based)**	
Meehan *et al*	7/17	2/16	4.9 (0.7–55.4)
Whatley *et al*	4/30	1/28	4.2 (0.4–212.0)
Total	11/47	3/44	4.6 (1.1–18.5)
Heterogeneity	Woolf Q = 0.01, df = 1, P = 0.9		
Overall effect	χ^2 = 4.6, df = 1, P = 0.03		

TEP = triethanolamine polypeptide, df = degrees of freedom.

Table 3 Effectiveness of preparations in facilitating successful syringing.

Study	Water-based	Oil-based	Odds ratio (95% CI)
Dubow	21/40	8/19	1.5 (0.4–5.3)
GP Research Group	39/47	48/60	1.2 (0.4–3.8)
Fraser	147/174	66/74	0.7 (0.2–1.6)
Chaput de Saintonge and Johnstone	21/35	20/32	0.9 (0.3–2.7)
Eekhof *et al*	21/22	19/20	1.1 (0.01–90.8)
Total	249/318	161/205	1.0 (0.6–1.6)
Heterogeneity	Woolf Q = 1.7, df = 4, P = 0.8		
Overall effect	χ^2 = 0.02 df = 1, P = 0.9		
	Docusate (water-based)	**TEP (water-based)**	
Fraser	23/26	19/24	2.0 (0.3–14.5)
Singer *et al*	17/23	6/21	7.1 (1.6–33.1)
Meehan *et al*	5/15	8/17	0.6 (0.1–2.9)
Whatley *et al*	18/34	13/30	(0.1–2.9)
Total	63/98	46/92	1.9 (0.7–5.0)
Heterogeneity	Woolf Q = 6.8, df = 3, P = 0.08		
Overall effect	χ^2 = 1.53, df = 1, P = 0.2		
	Docusate (water-based)	**Saline (water-based)**	
Meehan *et al*	5/15	8/16	0.5 (0.09–2.6)
Whatley *et al*	18/34	19/28	0.5 (0.2–1.7)
Total	23/49	27/44	0.5 (0.2–1.2)
Heterogeneity	Woolf Q = 0.004, df = 2, P = 0.9		
Overall effect	χ^2 = 2.3, df = 1, P = 0.1		
	TEP (water-based)	**Saline (water-based)**	
Meehan *et al*	8/17	8/16	0.9 (0.2–4.3)
Whatley *et al*	13/30	19/28	0.4 (0.1–1.2)
Total	21/47	27/44	0.5 (0.2–1.2)
Heterogeneity	Woolf Q = 1.0, df = 1, P = 0.3		
Overall effect	χ^2 = 2.35, df = 1, P = 0.1		
	Dioctyl (oil-based)	**Oil (oil-based)**	
GP Research Group	54/77	42/73	1.7 (0.8–3.6)
Burgess	19/34	33/41	0.3 (0.1–1.0)
Fraser	20/25	23/25	0.3 (0.03–2.5)
Total	93/136	98/139	0.6 (0.2 to 2.4)
Heterogeneity	Woolf Q = 9.0, df = 2, P = 0.01		
Overall effect	χ^2 = 0.5, df = 1, P = 0.5		

TEP = triethanolamine polypeptide, df = degrees of freedom.

Question 4

Julian, who is 15 years old and weighs 17 stone, tells you he has not been to school for 2 weeks and is contemplating suicide.

How would you manage this consultation? Discuss all relevant issues.

Question 5

Comment on the following, giving evidence to support your views:

a) Drug treatment of epilepsy

Comments	Evidence

b) Drug treatment of epilepsy in women on the pill and during pregnancy

Comments	Evidence

c) GP's role in diagnosis and monitoring of patients with epilepsy

Comments	Evidence

Question 6

One of the partners in your practice is under-performing—late for surgery, frequent sick leave, over-running, increased patient complaints, etc.

What issues does this raise in respect of:

a) The doctor

b) The patients

c) The partnership

d) How can this problem be addressed?

Question 7

Should there be an occupational health service for members of the primary health team? Discuss the advantages of such a service.

Question 8

Discuss the effectiveness of the following interventions in helping people to stop abusing alcohol:

a) Brief advice

b) Counselling

c) Alcohol detoxification services

d) Drug therapy

Question 9

Angela Jones comes to you to request a termination of pregnancy. She is 14 years old and does not want you to tell her parents. She tells you her boyfriend is 22.

Discuss all relevant issues.

Question 10

Billions of pounds are lost each year from incapacity benefit fraud and excessive sick notes. What is the GP's responsibility to society?

Discuss all relevant issues.

Question 11

Comment on the following medicolegal issues citing evidence to support your views:

a) Advance directives ('living will')

Comments	Evidence

b) Test of competency

Comments	Evidence

c) Confidentiality

Comments	Evidence

d) **Under-age consent**

Comments	Evidence

Question 12

Mrs Amy Johnson, a 35-year-old married woman, comes to your surgery and informs you that she is extremely depressed. She states that she has been tidying her affairs.

How do you manage this consultation?

Question 1: Answers

Your practice is planning a policy on prescribing antidepressants for depression.

Outline how you would gather your evidence.

- Determine target population. The management of depression in adolescents is controversial. Need to decide whether adolescents are to be treated with antidepressants by the GP or referred. The MHRA recommends that under 18s should not be prescribed SSRIs (except fluoxetine), as studies have shown increased suicidal and homicidal tendencies. Perhaps the practice policy should specify adults over the age of 18.
- Classify depression—mild, moderate, and severe.
- Consult the DSM-IV criteria for major depressive disorder, dysthymic disorder, and mild-to-moderate depression.
- Determine costs of each antidepressant and consider potential side-effects.
- Determine whether there is a gold standard of treatment. Access the Royal College of Psychiatry's website for the current management of depression. Access Medline and CINAHL for the most recent RCT studies.
- Consult *Clinical Evidence* on depressive disorders for the most recent advice and references. *Clinical Evidence* lists results of systematic reviews for the prescribing of antidepressants.
- Exclude non-randomised trials and those not pertinent to the UK.
- Consider use of a medical librarian to save on time gathering evidence.
- Define a time scale to devise this policy.
- Delegate duties to appropriate practice staff.
- Consult the National Research Register for any relevant ongoing studies.
- Consult local hospital psychiatric department for expert advice.
- Consult with pharmaceutical companies and read relevant drug bulletins.
- Consult the Medicines and Healthcare Products Regulatory Agency.
- Plan a practice meeting with all relevant parties and arrange follow-up for review after implementation. Consider audit.

Question 2: Answers

Your practice wishes to develop an evidence-based approach to the treatment of earwax.

a) **How would you ensure a comprehensive inclusion of studies?**

- I would ensure inclusion of all foreign as well as English literature to exclude publication bias.
- I would not be limited by time, i.e. not limit myself to current studies, to avoid bias introduced by a search limited to a particular period of time.
- I would use other search engines besides Medline to avoid database limitations.
- I would search the National Research Register to include ongoing studies.
- I would need to look at each study to match problem (trial size, participants' criteria, outcome measures, follow-up, randomisation, instruments, validity).
- One study that you discover is: The effectiveness of topical preparations for the treatment of earwax: a systematic review.

b) **The authors searched Medline. What are the strengths and weaknesses of Medline as a database?**

Strengths	Weaknesses
Efficient means of accessing huge database of articles and journals on world wide web	Limited by user's choice of search words. User bias
Able to select current review articles	Foreign articles are often excluded if not translated into English
	May not be able to obtain original article and have to settle for abstract instead so may influence choices
Able to select RCTs reviews	Bias introduced if other databases are not searched too
	Does not include ongoing studies. Excludes clinical experience and relies more on EBM

c) **Discuss the approach adopted by the authors to assess the evidence.**

- They chose to examine several databases instead of just Medline.
- They scrutinised the references of the review articles selected.
- They included ongoing studies.
- They accessed *Clinical Evidence* for the most recent advice.
- They contacted experts in the field who could speak from clinical experience.
- They excluded studies that were not randomised controlled studies.
- They chose to compare studies with similar outcome measures.

Question 3: Answers

Tables from the results section of the paper referred to in question 2 (The effectiveness of topical preparations for the treatment of earwax: a systematic review) are provided (please refer to **Reference material B**).

a)   **Interpret the results in Tables 2 and 3.**

Table 2

- The wide CI (0.2–27.2) in Singer *et al* suggests that the evidence is weak that docusate is more effective than TEP.
- However, pooling the three studies gave an OR of 0.8 with a CI of 0.2–2.8, suggesting that docusate is equally effective as TEP.
- Pooling the two studies comparing docusate with saline only showed weak evidence that docusate was more effective than saline with an OR of 1.9 and 95% CI of 0.4–8.8.
- Pooling the two studies comparing TEP with saline shows that TEP is more effective than normal saline (OR 4.6, 95% CI 1.1–18.5).

Table 3

- First study looks at five trials comparing water-based *vs* oil-based preparations in facilitating ear syringing. Pooling these data showed no statistical difference between use of water-based *vs* oil-based preps with an OR of 1 and a 95% CI of 0.6–1.6.
- Second study looks at four trials comparing docusate with TEP (both water-based preps). Pooling these data shows weak evidence that docusate is more effective than TEP (OR 1.9, 95% CI 0.7–5.0).
- Next two studies compared two trials looking at docusate *vs* saline and TEP *vs* saline and show weak evidence that saline is more effective than docusate or TEP.
- Last study looks at three trials comparing dioctyl (oil-based) with oil and pooling these data shows no difference in efficacy.

b)   **How might the evidence from Tables 2 and 3 influence your current practice?**

- Table 2 suggests that water-based docusate and TEP solutions are more effective than saline in clearing earwax. This suggests that I could prescribe colace or cerumenex. I would want to know if the studies were performed on children or adults and if the setting was an emergency department, ENT outpatient clinic, or GP setting.

- Table 3 suggests that there is no difference between water- and oil-based preps prior to ear syringing. It suggests that there is no reason to favour colace and cerumenex (water-based) over olive oil and cerumol (oil-based). The evidence is confusing when comparing Tables 2 and 3, as Table 2 suggests that docusate and TEP are more effective than saline and yet Table 3 suggests weak evidence to the contrary, i.e. that saline is more effective than docusate and TEP.

- I would also want to see the authors compare no treatment with water- or oil-based preps ± ear syringing.

- I am not convinced at this stage that I have enough information to make a decision to change my current practice of using sodium bicarbonate drops for cerumen.

Question 4: Answers

Julian, who is 15 years old and weighs 17 stone, tells you he has not been to school for 2 weeks and is contemplating suicide.

How would you manage this consultation? Discuss all relevant issues.

5000 people a year in the UK commit suicide and the group most at risk is young adult males under the age of 35. The NHS has stressed that it is committed to reducing this figure by 20% by the year 2010 according to the National Suicide Prevention Strategy for England.

Communication

- Sensitivity as Julian is a young teenager.
- Need to gain his trust.
- Need to come across as empathetic.
- Need to ask open-ended questions to encourage Julian to engage.
- Need to use open body language, non-threatening.
- Need to be consistent, parental role.

Issues for the patient

- Crisis point—call for help.
- Imminent danger of suicide.
- Depression.
- ? Substance abuse.
- ? Bullying.
- Weight issues.
- Low self-esteem.
- Family problems?

Issues for the GP

- Explore patient's ideas about suicide, concerns with weight, and expectations from GP.
- Dilemma for GP as patient has expressed an opinion for self-harm. Red flag GP notes and acknowledges that the consultation will run over time and therefore may wish to alert reception.

- Take history and perform mental and physical examination to exclude medical causes of obesity (diabetes, thyroid disease, endocrine disorders, etc), mental illness (depression, anxiety, victim of abuse by peers or family/close relatives), alcohol or drug abuse, etc.
- Ensure mental exam covers mood, loss of interest or pleasure, agitation, early morning wakening with rumination, impaired concentration, altered appetite, shame, guilt, suicide risk, substance abuse, and psychosis.
- Assess Julian's suicidal risk—plans? Past history of self-harm? Close relative has committed suicide? Assess mood stability.
- Assess Julian's support network. Abusive parents? Any close friends?
- Options for GP include watchful waiting, medication, counselling, CBT, referral to CMHT. GP needs to assess which option is viable here.
- May decide to contact rapid access psychiatric referral team and liaise with other agencies immediately.
- Assess involvement of other agencies—school reports, school attendance officers, school form teacher, social services involved with family, child at-risk register, educational welfare officers, past history of exclusion?
- GP needs to gain Julian's trust and confidence to ensure Julian will co-operate with management.
- ?Need for antidepressants but SSRIs are contraindicated in adolescents under the age of 18 so will need to consult psych team for opinion.
- Refer to practice counsellor—?need for long-term family counselling also.

Medicolegal issues

- Ensure patient confidentiality but may need to breach if deem patient is in imminent risk of suicide.
- Assess Fraser competence as Julian is under the age of 16 and if not competent, patient will need to have parent present.
- May decide Julian needs emergency sectioning under Section 4 of the Mental Health Act if he has made suicidal plans and refuses admission. Need to inform the parents.

Issues for the practice

- Ensure the practice is teenage-friendly with posters of teenagers on the wall, teenage magazines, teenage health leaflets, etc.
- Ensure the practice is teenage-sensitive with notices that ensure confidentiality to teenagers unless there is risk of harm to self or others.

Evidence

- 'Surviving Adolescence' mental health information on www.rcpsych.ac.uk.
- RCGP Adolescent Task Group www.rcgp.org.uk.
- DoH childhood obesity Sept 2003.
- NICE guideline: Management of depression in primary and secondary care, Dec 2003 www.nice.org.uk.
- NSF for mental health www.nehl.nhs.uk/nsf/mentalhealth/default.htm.
- National Suicide Prevention Strategy for England www.dh.gov.uk/asset Root/04/01/95/48/04019548.pdf.
- The International Statistical Classification of Diseases and Related Health Problems (ICD-10; WHO 1992).
- Criteria for Depressive Disorder DSM-IV. Diagnostic and Statistical Manual of Mental Disorders. The American Psychiatric Association.
- Committee on Safety of Medicines ban on paroxetine to under-18s. CSM review in December 2003 concluded that fluoxetine was the only drug in the class not linked to increased risk of self-harm and suicidal thoughts in adolescents. However, in the US, even fluoxetine is banned for the under-18s.

Question 5: Answers

Comment on the following, giving evidence to support your views:

a) **Drug treatment of epilepsy**

Comments	Evidence
First-line agent Sodium valproate (tonic-clonic fits, absence seizures, myoclonic jerks). Monitor for signs of blood or liver disorders, or pancreatitis	NICE guidelines 2004
First-line agent Carbamazepine (partial focal seizures ± secondary generalisation). Monitor for blood, liver, or skin disorders	NICE guidelines 2004
Oxycarbazepine (analogue of carbamazepine with less induction of hepatic enzymes). Avoid abrupt withdrawal	*British National Formulary*
Lamotrigine (monotherapy and adjunctive treatment of partial or generalised seizures). Be wary for rash in children or signs of bone marrow failure. Need to monitor hepatic, renal, and clotting factors	*British National Formulary*
Topiramate (adjunctive therapy for unresponsive seizure types)	*British National Formulary*
Vigabatrin (adjunct therapy for partial epilepsy). Monitor for visual field defects	*British National Formulary*
Phenytoin and phenobarbitone (older broad-spectrum drugs with sedative and drug interactions—not popular)	*British National Formulary*
Clonazepam (broad-spectrum agent for myoclonic jerks)	*British National Formulary*
Ethosuximide (absence seizures in children)	*British National Formulary*
Gabapentin (well-tolerated adjunctive therapy for partial epilepsy)	*British National Formulary*
Treatment cessation is only advised if the patient has been seizure-free for 2 years	

b) **Drug treatment of epilepsy in women on the pill and during pregnancy**

Comments	Evidence
Avoid hepatic enzyme inducers (carbamazepine, oxycarbazepine, phenytoin, phenobarbital, and topiramate) in patients on COC/POP. Offer depo-provera with injection intervals of 10 weeks instead of 12 or offer non-hormonal IUD	*British National Formulary*
Avoid carbamazepine, phenytoin, sodium valproate, which have been shown to be linked with neural tube defects	
Prescribe 5 mg folic acid daily preconceptually and during the first trimester	
Recommend use lamotrigine or gabapentin which are not known to be teratogenic	
Advise vitamin K1 prophylaxis against haemorrhagic disease of the newborn for women taking enzyme-inducing antiepileptics in the last month of pregnancy	

c) **GP role in diagnosis and monitoring of patients with epilepsy**

Comments	Evidence
GPs to refer patients within 2 weeks after first suspected epileptic seizure. Early referral is important as 15–30% of patients are misdiagnosed	NICE epilepsy guidelines 2004
RCTs show that immediate treatment of a single seizure with antiepileptic drug reduces seizure recurrence at 2 years compared with no treatment	*Clinical Evidence 2004*
GPs should perform annual reviews of all adult patients with well-controlled epilepsy. This entails tailoring treatment options and discussing lifestyle issues, such as ban on driving until fit-free for 12 months, childcare issues, etc. Refer patient to epilepsy specialist nurse. Children should be referred for annual review by a specialist	NSF guidelines for chronic conditions

Question 6: Answers

One of the partners in your practice is under-performing—late for surgery, frequent sick leave, over-running, increased number of errors, etc.

What issues does this raise in respect of:

a) **The doctor**

- Does the doctor have insight into the problem?
- Is he/she suffering from burnout?
- Does he/she have communication problems? Time management issues?
- Is there a source for his/her stress? Does he/she have personal, marital, or family problems? Recent bereavement? Does he/she have legal or financial burdens? Is he/she under litigation?
- Is he/she suffering from depression? Is he/she at risk of suicide? Does he/she have a mental illness?
- Does he/she have a substance misuse problem?
- Doctor is obliged not to work under the GMC's Fitness to Practise procedures if he/she feels his/her health is putting patients at risk.

b) **The patients**

- Concern over the continuity of care for his/her patients if the practice employs various locums to cover his/her sessions.
- Concern over chronic management of his/her patients if he/she is absent.
- Patients may be genuinely concerned over the health of their GP if he/she is well liked and this behaviour is unusual for him/her.
- Other partners may need to work extra sessions to cover his/her patients and this may lead to resentment.
- Patients' safety is at risk if he/she continues to work and is unfit.

c) **The partnership**

- What are the arrangements under the practice agreement with regard to sick leave? Extended time off for sabbatical (rest)? May need to employ a 6-month long-term locum.
- What are the doctor's obligations under the partnership agreement? Perhaps he/she should request a sabbatical? He/she needs to seek help.
- How do the other partners feel about putting in over-time to cover this GP's duties?
- Practice is at risk of litigation if the doctor continues to work and makes mistakes.

- Doctors are obliged to act under the Whistleblower's Act if they suspect a colleague is endangering the safety of patients but there is a due process—practice meeting, then LMC, then GMC.
- Doctors may consider seeking medicolegal advice from their medicolegal defence union, the BMA, the local PCT advisor.
- Doctors need to sit down with the colleague and ascertain why he/she is under-performing. Perform a preliminary assessment of his/her performance.

d) **How can this problem be addressed?**

- Take the colleague to one side and determine whether he/she has insight and is actively seeking help.
- Suggest the Sick Doctors Trust or National Counselling Service for Sick Doctors.
- Suggest the GP consults with his/her own GP for mental and physical health assessment.
- Suggest the GP takes extended sick leave so the practice can hire a 3–6 month locum to save on time and expense paying for ad-hoc locums and ensure safety of patients while he/she is seeking help.
- Need to be sensitive but also will need to notify GMC if the doctor refuses to comply and continues to put patients at risk.
- If the GP has an alcohol or drug misuse problem, the doctor should see his/her GP and be referred to the appropriate drug and alcohol management team. The doctor should be suspended from duties immediately and while undergoing treatment.

Evidence

- GMC Fitness to practise procedures: http://www.gmc-uk.org/
- The Sick Doctors Trust: http://www.sick-doctors-trust.co.uk/
- National Counselling Service for Sick Doctors: http://www.ncssd.org.uk

Question 7: Answers

Should there be an occupational health service for members of the primary health team? Discuss the advantages of such a service.

Yes, and as of April 2003, all PCOs have been obliged to provide occupational health services to the primary health service.

Why?

- GPs have a high incidence of suicide, depression, substance misuse, and stress/burnout.
- Primary health team is at risk from abuse from the public and from potential needle-stick injuries.
- Occupational health service can provide clinical staff with hepatitis B immunisation, Heaf test, and annual flu jabs.
- It can limit time taken off sick by offering a more accessible service than an employee's registered GP.
- Occupational health service can offer clinical advice on the management of needlestick injuries.
- It can refer or treat staff for counselling or physiotherapy.
- It can offer advice on ergonomics and VDU hazards.
- It can advise practices on the health and safety at work legislation regarding their responsibility to ensure the health and safety of all their employees and visitors to their premises.
- Service can manage sick doctors.
- Service can manage staff sick leave.
- Service can offer pre-employment screening.
- Service can suggest tips on dealing with stress, abusive patients, depression, hazards in the workplace, etc.

How?

- Funding to set up an occupational health service should be determined by the PCO or PCT as part of its mandatory obligation.
- Confidentiality of staff seen should be maintained at all times.
- Will attendance be deemed as compulsory or voluntary? For instance, should all clinical staff undergo a pre-employment screen?
- Who will monitor the quality of this service?
- Which staff are eligible for this service?
- Need to hire occupational health doctors and nurses. PCO will need to provide continued funding for staff and maintenance.

Question 8: Answers

Discuss the effectiveness of the following interventions in helping people to stop abusing alcohol:

a) **Brief advice**

- According to Wilson A, McDonald P, et al. Health promotion in the general practice consultation: a minute makes a difference. *BMJ* 1992 Jan;304:227–230, using a minute of a 10-min consultation to discuss alcohol use encourages patients to be forthcoming about their alcohol consumption.
- Brief intervention guidelines. Alcohol Concern, 1997.
- Edwards G, Marshall J, Cook C. *The Treatment of Drinking Problems. A Guide for the Helping Professionals*, 3rd edn. Cambridge: Cambridge University Press, 1997.

b) **Counselling**

- Alcoholics Anonymous meetings are an integral part of an initial treatment programme and are recommended by the Orange Book: *DoH's Drug Misuse and Dependence—Guidelines on Clinical Management.*
- Individual *vs* group counselling?

c) **Alcohol detoxification services**

- Outpatient alcohol detoxification is often sufficient according to the Orange Book and Collins MN, Burns T, van den Berk PA, Tubman GF. A structured programme for outpatient alcohol detoxification. *Br J Psychiatry* 1990 Jun;156:871–874. However, the following criteria must apply:
  — no history of delirium tremens or fits
  — no risk of suicide
  — social support available
  — no significant polydrug misuse
  — no benzodiazepine dependence.
- Inpatient alcohol detoxification with access to acute medical care is advocated by the Orange Book and combines use of tapering doses of librium or diazepam with group counselling. However, these forms of detoxification are no guarantee against relapse and therefore the patient must be aware that they have a chronic illness and constant effort is required on their part.

d) **Drug therapy**

- Disulfiram (Antabuse) is effective in helping patients maintain abstinence and may be offered to patients who have undergone detoxification and would like to remain alcohol free. According to the *British National Formulary*, it relies on inducing unpleasant systemic reactions when taken with alcohol, such as nausea, vomiting, headaches, flushing, because it leads to the accumulation of acetaldehyde. Excess alcohol consumption may lead to hypotension, arrhythmias, and collapse, and therefore this drug requires careful monitoring. Doses are commenced at 800 mg od and reduced over 5 days to 200 mg daily.
- Acamprosate may be used as an anticraving agent to maintain abstinence and may be used in combination with counselling.
- Long-acting benzodiazepines for a limited period to attenuate withdrawal symptoms and avoid dependence on benzos. Chlordiazepoxide (librium) is the drug of choice for detoxification according to the Orange Book and the dose and length of treatment depend on the severity of alcohol dependence. Starting dose may be 20–30 mg qds tapered to 10 mg nocte over 7 days. An alternate benzodiazepine is diazepam, which is used in inpatient detoxification centres.
- Chlormethiazole should be used for the management of withdrawal strictly in an inpatient setting.
- Vitamin B—oral vitamin B complex or vitamin B1 (thiamine) 50 mg bd should be prescribed for 3 weeks. For those with signs of Wernicke's encephalopathy or Korsakoff's psychosis, IV or IM administration of thiamine may be required.

Question 9: Answers

Angela Jones comes to you to request a termination of pregnancy. She is 14 years old and does not want you to tell her parents. She tells you her boyfriend is 22.

Discuss all relevant issues.

Issues for the patient

- Confidentiality.
- Autonomy.
- Fear of parents' wrath.
- Support network?
- Sensitive issue, embarrassment.
- *ICE*: Explore her ideas, concerns, and expectations with being pregnant and desiring a termination; also, was this rape?

Issues for the GP

- *Need to assess for competence.* A guidance report entitled *Confidentiality and People Under 16* issued by the BMA, GMSC, HEA, Brook Advisory Centres, FPA, and RCGP gives a step-by-step approach to this important ethical issue. The GP needs to assess her for 'Fraser competence' to consent to treatment. Competence is determined in terms of the patient's ability to understand the choices and their consequences, including the nature, purpose, and possible risks of any treatment (or non-treatment). The legal position dictates that the GP needs to determine whether the patient understands the potential risks and benefits of the treatment and the advice given.

  If the GP deems the patient to be 'Fraser competent', then she may give consent to a termination of pregnancy despite being under 16, and the GP may proceed without parental authority if satisfied that it is in her best interests. However, he/she may also consult the hospital obstetrician/gynaecologist for a second opinion if he/she cannot reach the conclusion that she is Fraser competent or that it is in her best interests.

- *Confidentiality.* The GP needs to stress at all times the value of parental support and explore reasons why the patient is unwilling to inform her parents. The GP should advise the patient that he/she is respecting her confidentiality. If the GP breaches confidentiality, he/she may jeopardise future trust. As Angela has disclosed the age of the father, the GP is obliged to breach confidentiality and inform the child protection agencies. He/she needs to inform Angela of his/her actions. He/she may wish to consult the MDU for confirmation.

- *Self-awareness.* The GP must acknowledge his/her own views/biases on abortion and under-age sex. He/she may even have a daughter of the same age.
- *Termination of pregnancy.* The GP should consult Angela's parents and obtain their written consent, unless she forbids the GP. Under the Abortion Act (1967), amended by the Human Fertilisation and Embryology Act (1990), there is no age limit. Instead, the GP needs to take into account whether her physical and/or mental health are likely to suffer if she does not undergo a termination of pregnancy, and must consider whether the patient's best interests require referral for termination of pregnancy to be with or without parental consent. The GP may consult the hospital for a second opinion as to whether this is in the patient's best interests and the matter may be referred to court for an order if he/she deems her Fraser incompetent and she refuses parental involvement.

   The GP also needs to assess gestation as this is a concealed pregnancy. If Angela is unsure of dates, the GP should palpate the abdomen and arrange an urgent dating scan.
- *Under-age sex ± consent, rape.* As she has disclosed that her male partner is 22, the GP is legally bound to report any under-age sex with an older man to the police. Duty of care and responsibility to society, as this is a question of rape under the law. The GP must inform the child protection agency. Reporting to social services under local child protection procedures will lead to liability to prosecution for the father of the baby under the Sexual Offences Act 2003.

Issues for the practice

- Ensure teenagers have access to contraceptive advice and methods if deemed Fraser competent.
- Teenage-friendly surgery—magazines, posters.
- Stress to teenagers the importance of using condoms and regular contraception if sexually active.
- Leaflets available to teens on local Brook Advisory Centres.
- Documentation in case of medicolegal action.
- Practice policy with respect to teenage issues.

Follow-up

- *Contraception/STDs.* If Angela decides to remain sexually active, she will need to be offered regular contraception. Various options in contraception should be discussed and user-friendly leaflets should be given to her to read. In surgery, the GP should take a full history to assess for contraindications, check her BP and weight, and advise her to commence regular contraception on day 1 of her next period. If she undergoes a TOP, discuss the option of a depo injection postop. If she opts for the pill, advice on missed pills, concurrent antibiotics, diarrhoea or vomiting, and potential side-effects should be discussed.

The GP should also offer STD screening as Angela has had UPSI and advise the use of condoms to protect herself from sexually transmitted diseases.

Question 10: Answers

Billions of pounds are lost each year from incapacity benefit fraud and excessive sick notes. What is the GP's responsibility to society?

Discuss all relevant issues.

Issues for the GP

- Fear of retaliation or reprisal from patients for sick note refusal.
- Personal view that it is not the GP's responsibility to police patients.
- Time constraints may influence the GP to issue a certificate rather than discuss with the patient why he/she should go back to work.
- GP's role is as patient advocate. There is a conflict of interest in both patient care and relationship.
- GP cannot effectively dispute a patient's claim of stress, depression, or chronic low back pain on history or examination. Patient usually presents with a convincing story.
- Often patients assume, wrongly, that it is their right to receive a sick certificate from their GP whenever they want.

Issues for the practice

- Patients may become hostile to staff and upset patients in the waiting room if refused a sick certificate.
- Patients may put in undue complaints against GPs if refused.
- Practice should advise patients that for the first 4 days of sickness they do not require a sick note. For the next 3 days off sick, they are obliged to complete a self-certificate-2 from the employer and not request one from the GP until >7 days have been taken off sick.
- Practice can print a leaflet for patients with regards to the sick note policy. This should also cover private sick notes and patients should be informed of the practice fee for these.

Wider issues

- Consider a policy authorising practice nurses to write sick notes instead?
- NHS hospital trusts—integration of sickness certificates into discharge procedures (Regulatory Impact Unit—*Making a Difference*, GP Report, June 2002 www.cabinet-office.gov.uk/regulation).

- Employers should be encouraged to offer SC-2 forms for 7 days to employees instead of insisting on a doctor's note.
- Government should take away the onerous task of sick notes from GPs, as not all GPs are trained in occupational health to be competent to assess a patient's ability to work. This task should be left to the company doctor, outside occupational health agency, or DoH.
- At present, patients who take >4 months off sick are referred to occupational health. This length of time should be reduced to take the burden off GPs. The RM-7 form does, however, allow GPs to question whether a patient is malingering and an independent medical reviewer will assess the patient asking for repeated med3 certs.
- Government or employing bodies should introduce financial incentives for employees to remain healthy and limit sick leave.
- Government should reduce the financial compensation for sick pay, so that it is not profitable to remain off sick for a lengthy period.
- Government should institute a policy whereby an employer may make an employee redundant if he/she takes >1 month off sick per year to encourage small businesses to thrive and to discourage fraud. However, this is a contentious topic and may be influenced by the political agenda of the government in office.

Question 11: Answers

Comment on the following medicolegal issues citing evidence to support your views:

a) **Advance directives ('living will')**

Comments	Evidence
Patient issues: need to obtain templates. If the living will just states DNR or is 10 years old, it can be deemed invalid. Better to be written, dated, witnessed, specific to the condition, and regularly updated	Terence Higgins Trust The Voluntary Euthanasia Society
Doctor issues: need to establish if it is valid? Is it specific to this situation? What is in the best interest of the patient? (include medical prognosis, post-recovery state, future happiness, social issues, etc)	Guidelines by GMC and BMA
Doctor issues: need to inform secondary services after establishing validity of will	

b) **Test of competency**

Comments	Evidence
Legal test of competency states that the person be able to understand the facts presented and to weigh them up in a decision-making process	BMA, GMC, English law
Doctor issues: this may guide a doctor when assessing elderly patients with dementia or establishing Fraser competence in an under 16 yo patient to detemine whether he/she is competent to receive or refuse treatment	

c) **Confidentiality**

Comments	Evidence
Patient issues: 'It is not an absolute right. It is a qualified right.' The right of respect for a private and family life.	Human Rights Act (1998)
Doctor has the right to breach confidentiality if there is risk of harm to person or society	Article 8 subsection 1 of the Human Rights Act (1998)
Doctor issues: he/she must not breach a patient's qualified right to confidentiality, unless it is an important issue (rape, murder), for which the patient's right to confidentiality is waived for the benefit of society	Case of Z vs Finland

d) **Under-age consent**

Comments	Evidence
Consent must be given by parent(s) for children aged under 18	Children's Act (1989)
Only in respect of medical treatment can a person of 16 or over give consent. Said person is given autonomy of decision-making	Family Law Reform Act (1969)
Under 16s if deemed Gillick (Fraser) competent are competent to give consent	Gillick vs West Norfolk Health Authority
Patient issues: under 16s if deemed Fraser competent may obtain contraception and request TOP, i.e. are fully autonomous in medical matters	GMC, BMA, MPS, MDU
Doctor issues: need to assess Fraser competency in under 16s but may be able to resort to secondary services, i.e. consultant obstetrician, court, to obtain a second opinion if in doubt about child's competency	GMC, BMA, MPS, MDU

Question 12: Answers

Mrs Amy Johnson, a 35-year-old married woman, comes to your surgery and informs you that she is extremely depressed. She states that she has been tidying her affairs.

How do you manage this consultation?

Issues for the patient

- Asking for help.
- Sense of hopelessness, helplessness, despondency. Loss of control.
- Embarrassment, stigma of mental illness
- Marital strife—separation or divorce?
- Financial debts?
- Chronic illness?
- Occupational problems—bullying?
- Recent bereavement or suicide by relative or close friend?

Issues for the doctor

- Assess depression. How is her appetite, sleep, mood, enjoyment of interests, support network? Has she been on antidepressants?
- Assess immediate risk of suicide. The cue is that she has told the doctor that she is tidying her affairs. This is an important cue that she is contemplating ending her life. Conduct a full history. Are there any triggers—work, home, mental or physical illnesses, bereavements, or financial problems? Has she made plans? Has a family member committed suicide in the past or recently? Has she had any life traumas—childhood abuse, rape? Does she see a future?
- Have a low threshold for contacting the Rapid Access Psychiatric Team or admitting her to a psychiatric ward if you are not entirely convinced that she is safe. Remember 80% of women see a health professional prior to committing suicide.
- How old are the children? Do they need to be put on the children at-risk register? Does Amy have a prior history of suicide attempts? How aware are the children?
- Self-awareness—time constraint, running late. However, acknowledge that this consultation is a 'life or death' visit and takes utmost priority.
- Self-awareness—of own views on suicide. Be non-judgemental.

- If entirely convinced that she is safe, discuss options of counselling, anti-depressants, and close monitoring at the surgery. Be wary of starting SSRIs, which are known to increase agitation and suicidal tendencies. If commenced, add an antianxiolytic and monitor patient on a weekly basis to exclude increased suicidal risk and warn Amy. Drug options also include SNRIs, e.g. venlafaxine, which is now first-line with many psychiatrists.

Evidence-based medicine

- Of the 140,000 who attempt suicide each year in England and Wales, one in five will make a further attempt, of which 10% will be fatal. Attempted suicide is therefore a risk factor. There are calls for 'improvement to risk management skills, recognition and management of depression, and recognition of suicide risk.' *National Suicide Prevention Strategy for England.* London: DoH, 2002.
- 80% of women, 50% of men aged 25 and over, and 20% of men aged <25 see a health-care professional prior to committing suicide. Pirkis J, Burgess P. Suicide and recency of health care contacts. *Br J Psychiatry* 1998 Dec;173:462–474.
- Risk factors include relationship and occupational problems, psychological trauma, violence, and psychiatric illness (bipolar, depression, schizophrenia), chronic illness, increasing age, social isolation, male gender, and race, cultural or sexuality issues. Mood disorders and suicide. *J Clin Psychiatry* 2001;27–30.
- Predictors of suicide risk include past attempts within the last 12 months, the suicide of a close relative, tidying up personal affairs, taking out a life insurance policy, making a will, and change in behaviour (low mood or excessively high mood). Practice guideline for the assessment and treatment of patients with suicidal behaviors. *Am J Psychiatry* 2003 Apr;160:1–60.
- Strategy to reduce morbidity and mortality due to suicidal behaviour. *SUPRE, The Worldwide Initiative for the Prevention of Suicide.* Geneva: WHO, 2004.

Written Paper Three

For the Royal College of General Practitioners' Instructions and Glossary for the Written Paper Module, see pages 18–19

Question 1

Mr Mark Kingsley tells you that he would like to make a complaint against you for refusing to visit his 40-year-old wife who is at home with flu.

Discuss all pertinent issues.

Question 2

Please read the extract from the paper entitled: Population based randomised controlled trial on impact of screening on mortality from abdominal aortic aneurysm (please refer to **Reference material A**) and answer the question given below.

Comment on the strengths and weaknesses of the methodology of the study population for this study.

Reference Material A
(Question 2)

Population based randomised controlled trial on impact of screening on mortality from abdominal aortic aneurysm.
Norman PE, Jamrozik K, Lawrence-Brown MM, *et al.*
BMJ *2004 Nov;*329:1259–1262.

Methods

Study population
To provide the most rigorous possible test of the utility of screening, the authors designed the trial as a population-based study with the primary end point, mortality from abdominal aortic aneurysm, to be analysed on an intention to treat basis. The authors planned to have 90% power to detect and declare significant (two-sided $\alpha = 0.05$) a relative reduction of 50% in mortality among men invited for screening over 5 years from the start of screening. Using available pilot data, the authors estimated that the control group would need to contain about 20,000 men to experience 55 deaths from abdominal aortic aneurysm.

Men were identified from an electronic copy of the electoral roll, enrolment to vote being compulsory for all Australian adults. At the beginning of the trial the authors selected all 41,000 men on the electoral roll who were resident to Perth and were expected to be 65–79 years old at the projected mid-point of screening. Men were randomised into intervention and control groups of equal size defined by 5-year group and postcode. Men in the control group were allocated a 'virtual' date of screening, which was the median scheduled date of examination for men from the same postcode area randomised to the intervention group. Men in the intervention group were sent a letter explaining the study and offering an appointment for a scan. Men who did not take up the initial invitation to screening were sent a second letter.

At the five screening clinics the greatest transverse and anteroposterior diameter was measured with a Toshiba Capasee ultrasound machine with a 3.75 MHz probe. On leaving the clinic, each man was given a letter containing results of his scan, with a copy for his GP. The GP arranged any follow-up investigations or referral to a surgeon. The authors made no attempt to influence any aspects of clinical management, in particular with regard to threshold for intervention or method of repair.

Question 3

Tables from the results section of the paper referred to in question 2 (Population based randomised controlled trial on impact of screening on mortality from abdominal aortic aneurysm) are provided (please refer to **Reference material B**).

a) **Interpret the results in Tables 2 and 3.**

b) **How might the evidence from Tables 2 and 3 influence your current practice?**

Reference Material B
(Question 3)

Population based randomised controlled trial on impact of screening on mortality from abdominal aortic aneurysm.
Norman PE, Jamrozik K, Lawrence-Brown MM, *et al*.
BMJ *2004 Nov*;329:1259–1262.

Reproduced with permission from the BMJ Publishing Group.

Table 2 Elective and emergency procedures and crude and age-standardised mortality from abdominal aortic aneurysm between scheduled screening and the end of follow-up.

	Elective		Emergency					
	Operation	Postop deaths (%)	All ruptures	Ops ruptures	Postop deaths	Fatal rupture without surg	Total (%)	Age-standardised mortality (95% CI)
Intervention group								
Scanned (n=12,203)	86	4 (4.7)	3	0	0	3	7(0.06)	7.8 (1.91–13.05)
Not scanned (n=7149)	21	0	30	9	1	10	11(0.15)	18.27 (7.08–29.46)
Total invited (n=19,352)	107	4 (3.7)	33	9	1	13	18(0.09)	11.51 (6.16–16.86)
Control group								
Total invited (n=19,352)	54	3 (5.6)	38	8	3	19	25(0.13)	18.91 (10.97–26.85)

Table 3 Elective and emergency procedures, deaths, and crude and age-standardised mortality from abdominal aortic aneurysm between randomisation and the end of follow-up.

	Elective		Emergency					
	Operation	Postop deaths (%)	All ruptures	Ops ruptures	Postop deaths	Fatal rupture without surg	Total (%)	Age-standardised mortality (95% CI)
Intervention group								
Scanned (n=12,203)	86	4 (4.7)	3	0	0	3	7 (0.06)	7.8 (1.91 to 13.05)
Not scanned (n=8297)	26	1 (3.9)	35	11	2	21	24 (0.29)	46.56 (24.7 to 68.4)
Total invited (n=20,500)	112	5 (4.5)	38	11	2	24	31 (0.15)	23.55 (13.79 to 33.31)
Control group								
Total invited (n=20,500)	60	4 (6.7)	41	10	5	28	37 (0.18)	27.83 (16.89 to 38.77)

Question 4

Comment on the value of the following, giving evidence to support your views:

a) Antiarrhythmic drugs for atrial fibrillation

Comments	Evidence

b) Rate-controlling drugs for atrial fibrillation

Comments	Evidence

c) Anticoagulation therapy for atrial fibrillation

Comments	Evidence

d) **Ablation therapy for atrial fibrillation**

Comments	Evidence

Question 5

You have been informed that your patient has just committed suicide from an overdose of co-proxamol. You had commenced her on prozac 3 weeks earlier.

Discuss a 'significant event analysis' of this incident in terms of process, prevention, and possible outcomes.

Question 6

Your partner requests a 6-month sabbatical.

Discuss all relevant issues.

Question 7

Dr Des Spence of No Free Lunch states that drug reps do influence GPs' prescribing patterns and should be banned. He suggests keeping a register of how many times a drug rep visits a surgery.

What issues does this raise?

Question 8

You find a half-empty bottle of whisky on your partner's desk and note that he smells of alcohol in the mornings.

How do you decide when to act?

Question 9

An 80-year-old patient tells you she would like to leave you personally £10,000 in her will.

What do you tell her?

Question 10

How would you go about setting up a practice protocol for telephone consultations?

Question 11

Comment on the management of the following skin conditions, giving evidence to support your views:

a) Acne

Comments	Evidence

b) Eczema (allergic, atopic, discoid, venous)

Comments	Evidence

c) Psoriasis

Comments	Evidence

d) **Fungal infections**

Comments	Evidence

Question 12

Mrs Fatima Khan, a 34-year-old woman, comes to your surgery and states that she has no interest in sex with her husband. She explains that she has pain during sexual intercourse since the birth of her first baby.

How do you manage this consultation?

Question 1: Answers

Mr Mark Kingsley tells you that he would like to make a complaint against you for refusing to visit his 40-year-old wife who is at home with flu.

Discuss all pertinent issues.

Communication issues

- Mr Kingsley is making an inappropriate request from you. However, try to use verbal and nonverbal forms of communication to appease him and try to explain why it is inappropriate for his wife to request a home visit for flu.
- Acknowledge that this is a dysfunctional consultation.
- Determine what Mr Kingsley had hoped to achieve by a home visit. What are his concerns?
- Suggest that he or a mini cab drive his wife to the practice for a complete history and examination. Try to gift-wrap the concept that a consultation at the practice is more beneficial for his wife as there you will have access to further investigations, etc, if deemed necessary.
- If he still wishes to complain, you are obliged to inform him of your inhouse complaints procedure which should conform to the national criteria as issued by the NHS Executive.
- Good communication drastically reduces the risk of complaints. (Beckman HB, et al. Arch Intern Med 1994;154:1365).

Patient issues

- Mr Kingsley may be under duress from his wife who may also have a hidden agenda. He may have had a bad day and is taking it out on you.
- Does he feel you are 'fobbing them off'?
- Mrs Kingsley may have her own unrealistic ideas and expectations of the role of a GP.
- Mr and Mrs Kingsley may be convinced in their minds that the GP is at fault and blow the situation out of proportion. They may become hostile to the GP and this will jeopardise future patient–doctor care and trust.

Doctor issues

- Self-awareness of complaints as a severe source of stress in the work place. An Australian study showed that for GPs the threat of litigation was the most severe source of stress. (www.medicine.au.net.au/columns/legal/lega246.html)
- Number of complaints against GPs doubled in 1998 following a change to the NHS complaints procedure in 1996. The latter was made from recommendations in the 1994 Wilson Report.
- Individual reaction—depending on personality type, a complaint may impact on a GP's personal life and self-esteem. He/she may feel isolated and depressed. He/she must seek support.
- GP is aware that he/she must try to resolve the matter in his/her consultation, i.e. prevention of a complaint is desirable, but if unable to, then he/she must inform the patient of the inhouse complaints procedure. Patient must complete a complaints form for the practice manager. Patient's rights to confidentiality will be observed. An appointment will be made for the complainant with the practice manager. A letter of acknowledgement will be sent to him/her within 2 working days. Practice manager will undertake investigation of the complaint and will ask the GP to respond in writing. Findings will then be discussed in a partners' meeting and a letter will be sent to the complainant within 10 working days.
- GP may feel that in future his/her consultations need to be more patient-centred to avoid complaints. However, there is a risk when the consultation is skewed too far towards the patient.

Medicolegal issues

- If complaint fails to be resolved at practice level, complainant may ask for an independent review from the local PCT.
- Role of the PCT is to do nothing if the complaint has been addressed appropriately; to refer back to the practice level; to organise conciliation; to set up an independent review panel; or to advise complainant of his/her right to approach the Health Service Ombudsman.
- Disciplinary panels may be set up by the PCT or referral made to the GMC if there is concern regarding a GP's Fitness to Practise for medical reasons, allegations of serious professional misconduct, or evidence of severely deficient professional performance.

Evidence

- Medical Defence Union. *Problems in General Practice: Complaints and How to Avoid Them.* MDU, 1996.

Question 2: Answers

Please read the extract from the paper entitled: Population based randomised controlled trial on impact of screening on mortality from abdominal aortic aneurysm (please refer to **Reference material A**) and answer the question given below.

Comment on the strengths and weaknesses of the methodology of the study population for this study.

Strengths

- Use of equal number of controls.
- Randomisation of intervention and control groups of equal size.
- Use of electoral roll to obtain a large sample representative of the population.
- Sample size is sufficient to detect significant statistical results.
- Power has been calculated.

Weaknesses

- Did not use general practice lists.
- Not representative of a UK population as study was based in Perth.
- The gold standard, i.e. the multicentre aneurysm screening study, looked at screening men between 65 and 74 years as having the potential to reduce mortality. The target age of 65–83 is too broad and introduces confounding factors, e.g. poor candidates for surgery, concomitant heart disease, etc.
- Did not exclude patients with co-morbidities, too ill, nursing home residents, etc; i.e. confounding factors will increase mortality in this age group.
- As patients were managed independently by GPs after the screening scan, the timing of referral for surgery was variable, which introduces bias.

Question 3: Answers

Tables from the results section of the paper referred to in question 2 (Population based randomised controlled trial on impact of screening on mortality from abdominal aortic aneurysm) are provided (please refer to **Reference material B**).

a) **Interpret the results in Tables 2 and 3.**

Table 2

- Table of the numbers of operations and deaths from AAA after screening.
- Overall mortality was 4.3% (7/161) after elective surgery and 24% (4/17) after emergency surgery for ruptured AAA.
- Twice as many men in the intervention group underwent surgery compared to the control group.
- 18 men died from AAA in the intervention group and 25 in the control group, which gives a mortality rate ratio of 0.61.
- No statistically-significant difference between the intervention group and control group.
- Suggests that a screening programme does not significantly reduce mortality in the 65–83-year age group.

Table 3

- Table of the corresponding numbers of operations and deaths from AAA between randomisation and the end of follow-up.
- Overall mortality was 5.2% (9/172) after elective surgery and 8.9% (7/79) after emergency surgery for ruptured AAA.
- Twice as many men in the intervention group underwent surgery compared to the control group.
- 31 men died from AAA in the intervention group and 37 in the control group, which gives a mortality ratio of 0.85.
- No statistically-significant difference in mortality between the intervention group and control group.
- Suggests that a screening programme does not significantly reduce mortality in the 65–83-year age group.

b) **How might the evidence from Tables 2 and 3 influence your current practice?**

There are too many confounding variables for this study to be valid. By inclusion of all men between 65 and 83 on the electoral roll, no selective exclusion of unfit candidates took place. Those too ill or with concomitant chronic illnesses would affect surgical morbidity and mortality. By having individual GPs decide on the criteria for referral of patients to the vascular surgeons, more bias was introduced. Therefore, this study would not change my practice.

Question 4: Answers

Comment on the value of the following, giving evidence to support your views:

a) **Antiarrhythmic drugs for atrial fibrillation**

Comments	Evidence
Flecainide and propafenone Contraindicated in IHD and impaired ventricular function as may cause arrhythmias	*British Heart Foundation Factfile*, Oct 2004 *Clinical Evidence*, June 2004 One RCT found that IV flecainide increased reversion to sinus rhythm within 1 h and maintained it after 6 h compared to placebo Three RCTs found no significant difference in rates of conversion to sinus rhythm between flecainide and propafenone
Dofetilide (beneficial in patients with impaired ventricular function)	*British Heart Foundation Factfile*, Oct 2004
Amiodarone (most effective agent but requires 6-monthly monitoring of LFTs and TFTs)	*British Heart Foundation Factfile*, Oct 2004

b) **Rate-controlling drugs for atrial fibrillation**

Comments	Evidence
Rate control strategy preferred over rhythm control	AFFIRM study. 4060 patients with AF were randomised to treatment with rate control *vs* rhythm control. More patients in the rhythm control group were hospitalised and had more adverse drug effects
Beta-blockers to maintain sinus rate. Safe treatment	*British Heart Foundation Factfile*, Oct 2004 *British National Formulary*
Digoxin reduces ventricular rate	*Clinical Evidence*, June 2004 Two RCTs showed that digoxin reduces ventricular rate after 30 min compared with placebo
Diltiazem	*Clinical Evidence*, June 2004 One RCT showed that IV diltiazem reduces ventricular rate in 15 min compared with placebo

c) **Anticoagulation therapy for atrial fibrillation**

Comments	Evidence
Warfarin anticoagulation is indicated for patients with AF + valvular disease	*British Heart Foundation Factfile,* Oct 2004
Warfarin anticoagulation is indicated for AF patients without valvular disease who have one or more of the following risk factors: age >65, previous embolic event(s), diabetes, or hypertension.	
Target INR is between 2 and 3. Monitor for risk of bleeding and dosage adjustment	
Ximelagatran (oral direct inhibitor of thrombin)	Due to be licensed in 2005 SPORTIF III trial compared this agent to warfarin in 3410 patients with AF and one or more stroke RFs. Similar benefits but ximelagatran was associated with fewer haemorrhages

d) **Ablation therapy for AF**

Comments	Evidence
Ablation of the pulmonary vein/left atrial border (site for initiation of AF) using radiofrequency energy has a 70% success rate but also carries a risk of cardiac tamponade	Jais P, et al. Ablation therapy for atrial fibrillation (AF): past, present and future. *Cardiovasc Res* 2002;54(2):337–346.
Ablation of the AV node/His bundle is catheter based and is effective in abolishing and reducing symptoms. It is a palliative measure and requires pacemaker implantation and further anticoagulation	*British Heart Foundation Factfile,* Oct 2004

Question 5: Answers

You have been informed that your patient has just committed suicide from an overdose of co-proxamol. You had commenced her on prozac 3 weeks earlier.

Discuss a 'significant event analysis' of this incident in terms of process, prevention, and possible outcomes.

Process

- The *SEA Guidelines for General Practice*, as issued by the Integrated GP Quality Group in August 2002, covers the process in detail. The process involves acknowledging that an event which is out of the ordinary has resulted in harm and there is a need to discuss this event bearing in mind the principles of a no-blame culture, a learning environment with protected time, and potential for change to improve care.
- A specified date, time, and place are arranged and a chairman is appointed to facilitate.
- A background SEA form is completed to gather evidence. This form should include a detailed description of the event (including past history of suicide attempts by the deceased patient or past history of suicide attempts in practice patients on prozac), name of the person reporting the event, people involved in the event and/or to be involved in the discussion, perceived problems, a list of outcomes and recommendations, areas of feasible improvement, and educational needs identified. How to meet the educational needs and how to demonstrate improvement need to be addressed.
- Aim of the SEA is to improve care.
- Discussion at the SEA meeting should be recorded by hand, and the discussion should encompass the background SEA and also all relevant issues raised by the event: what went well?; what went less well?; and how might we have done things differently?

Prevention

- SEA meeting should discuss important risk factors such as the patient's previous history of suicide attempts and if she was prescribed co-proxamol in the past so had access to it.
- Precautionary measures to prevent future added risk of suicide in patients should be identified and a discussion should take place on how these ele-

ments can be implemented. The number of co-proxamol tablets on a practice px could be limited to 12 to prevent accidental overdose. Patients who have a prior history of suicide attempts or suicidal ideation are unsuitable candidates for prozac. Patients should be warned that prozac increases suicidal tendencies and may cause intrusive suicidal thoughts. Patients may need weekly monitoring for this risk in the first month of use.

Outcomes of SEA

- Outcome should include identification of a wide variety of areas/needs for clinical improvement, educational needs, resource needs, and acquisition and audit needs. There should be mutual agreement for change and ongoing monitoring of this change.
- Wider issues might include a call for further investigation into the safety of SSRIs, increased patient awareness of the hazards of overdose on co-proxamol (detropropoxyphene is a derivative of morphine for which there is no antidote), and the potential hazards of SSRIs (increased agitation and increased suicidal tendencies). Local PCT could determine if there is a link in local practices between SSRIs and suicide and ask for a national investigation.

Further reading

- MacDonald L. *Significant Event Analysis Guidelines for General Practice.* Integrated General Practice Quality Group, August 2002.
- Rughani A. Significant event analysis. In: *The GP's Guide to Personal Development Plans*, 2nd edn. Oxford: Radcliffe Medical Press, 2001.

Question 6: Answers

Your partner requests a 6-month sabbatical.

Discuss all relevant issues.

Issues for the partner

- Why is he/she requesting a sabbatical? And why now? What are his/her ideas, concerns, and expectations from this 6-month sabbatical?
- Is he/she suffering burnout, stress, etc? What is his/her personal and family situation like?
- Is this a cry for help? Is he/she depressed over litigation or a recent crisis?

Issues for the patients

- Loss of continuity of care.
- May be genuinely concerned over the health of the partner.
- Increased time to get an appointment as the practice is now one GP down so the practice will not be able to reach its target of 48 h.
- Care of patients may be put at risk by overburdened partners. Increase in patient complaints? Increased mistakes?

Issues for the practice

- Financial implications of hiring a locum for 6 months and paying the partner's salary. Locums working 6 months are now entitled to 2 weeks' paid annual leave. Additional costs to bear and who will cover the locum's holiday? Advertising costs? Locums expect competitive rates of pay.
- What does it state in the partner's agreement regarding sabbatical leave?
- A request for leave does not ensure entitlement.
- Is this a soft way of leaving the practice? Will he/she return?
- Unhappy staff and an extra 2500 patients without a GP.
- Resentment among partners who may already feel burdened and stressed outside the workplace.
- How does the sabbatical benefit the practice? A practice meeting will need to be held with the partner in question, the practice manager, and the partners, and all relevant issues need to be addressed before reaching a decision.

Wider issues

- What is the policy regarding GP sabbaticals in the local surgeries or in a PCT? Is there uniformity? Is one practice more lenient than another? Need for equity.
- Is there a PCT policy regarding time permitted for sabbaticals?
- Should the PCT allow paid 6-month sabbaticals for GPs who have worked a decade or more and pay for the costs of a locum, as being a GP is a highly stressful job? This may be an incentive for GPs to stay in practice and a way out if feeling overburdened. Also, pursuing an outside interest is known to alleviate stress.

Question 7: Answers

Dr Des Spence of No Free Lunch states that drug reps do influence GPs' prescribing patterns and should be banned. He suggests keeping a register of how many times a drug rep visits a surgery.

What issues does this raise?

Issues for the drug reps

- Drug reps are being paid to increase GP awareness and increase market sales of their brand drug product over their competitors.
- Need to possess integrity and maintain trust of GP as they are in effect working colleagues.
- Large pharmaceutical companies have a larger budget for their drug reps to persuade GPs with freebies, free meals, free funding of away days, free catering for talks, etc. Smaller drug companies are at a disadvantage, which becomes an issue for the Monopolies Commission.

Issues for the doctor

- *Probity*: One of the codes of good medical practice is to be honest. Under the Health and Social Care Bill (2001), all gifts >£25 should be declared and all gifts >£100 should be registered for tax purposes. Freebie items such as pens and post-its can be declared in the practice log. Need to say 'No' to cash incentives. These may be seen as a bribe. May accept a free lunch or free pen but if feels uncomfortable with the level of gift, then should decline the gift or else may feel beholden to drug reps and this may influence decision-making when prescribing treatment.
- *Providing good clinical care*: GP needs to be aware when listening to information regarding a new drug product that drug reps are biased. GP needs to make his/her own decisions by weighing up all the facts from the drug reps, colleagues, hospital consultants, evidence-based medicine, peer-reviewed journals, NICE, WHO and royal college guidelines.
- *Equity*: GP has a budget for prescribing and therefore should prescribe generic drugs that are effective and not rely on expensive drugs if they are only equally as effective. Concern arises if GP is faced with a dilemma—a more expensive alternative which has been proven to be more beneficial to the patient. The GP is aware of his/her annual PACT statement and may feel pressured to prescribe the cheaper, less effective drug to stay within

budget, which may ultimately not be the best care of the patient. Alternatively, he/she may feel he/she needs to prescribe the more expensive drug because it is more effective for the patient.

Issues for the patient

- Patients want the best drug available but are unaware of the cost issue. They often come as consumers. Drug reps can inform GP of new and expensive drugs but GP must decide whether they truly are more beneficial to the patient and examine the drug profile with due diligence.
- Patient only wants a drug that works now and has few or no side-effects. The patient is more concerned with the theory of right *vs* the theory of utility.

Wider issues

- Currently, a health review board is examining the role of drug reps and whether they influence GPs in their choices of prescriptions.
- The Association of the British Pharmaceutical Company, based in Whitehall, has a trade standards department that is alerted to illegal practices by pharma companies and will investigate and stop such practices, e.g. paid weekend holidays, daily visits by drug reps (average should be three times a year), etc.
- Safety-net. PCT issues an annual PACT statement to each practice detailing percentage of generic *vs* brand-name prescribing, annual expenditures, categorises prescriptions, and compares practices in the PCT. It becomes apparent if one practice is over-prescribing brand-name drugs and the PCT will send a prescribing advisor to that practice to look into the matter.

Question 8: **Answers**

You find a half-empty bottle of whisky on your partner's desk and note that he/she smells of alcohol in the mornings.

How do you decide when to act?

Issues for the doctor

- Need to be sensitive to your partner.
- Need to gather hard evidence and not rely solely on circumstantial evidence.
- Need to assess whether the partner is putting patients at risk. Is he/she fit to practise? Good medical practice suggests that if a colleague is putting patients at risk, he/she should suspend duties immediately.
- As suspicion has been aroused, action needs to be taken now to arrange for a preliminary evaluation of the partner's performance by assessing his/her Fitness to Practise in terms of Good Medical Practice.
- Is he/she providing good clinical care?
- Is he/she maintaining good medical practice (keeping up to date, good audit results, average referral rates, PACT data?). Bear in mind that this criterion has its limits, e.g. a GP with specialist training may refer more as he/she will know more about the range of available specialist services, which does not in itself indicate he/she is a poorly performing GP. Alternatively, a GP who prescribes expensive drugs may have more expert knowledge of a condition and know that drug X is more efficacious with fewer side-effects. However, collectively, the evidence should paint a more realistic picture.
- Does he/she show respect and obtain consent from his/her patients (no patient complaints, good patient satisfaction surveys)?
- Does he/she work well with colleagues and staff (tardiness, rude?, practice staff's opinion)?
- Are his/her annual appraisals up to date?
- Does he/she have insight into his/her own health?
- Is he/she honest about doubts of probity—records honest and above scrutiny?
- May use quality markers to assess GP also.

Issues for the partner

- Need to respect Beauchamps and Childress' four principles of ethics.
- Respect partner's autonomy. Sit down with the partner and gather information. Any particular personal or family stresses? How much is he/she drinking?
- Ensure beneficence and no harm to his/her patients. Suspend duties of the doctor immediately if suspicions are confirmed.
- Respect partner's confidentiality but may breach if putting patients at risk as per Article 8 subsection 1 of the Human Rights Act.
- Ensure equity of treatment for all poorly performing GPs. Do not become judgmental and whistle-blow immediately to the GMC. Be sensitive and understanding and offer due process—informal meeting, then formal practice meeting, then refer up to the LMC, then the GMC if the matter fails to be resolved along the way.

Issues for the practice

- Need to call for a practice meeting with all relevant clinical staff and the partner in question.
- Need to gather evidence from staff and patients as to whether the partner is jeopardising the care of patients.
- Need to have a plan of action, e.g. suspend duties of the doctor while he is obtaining help from AA and a detox programme.
- Financial costs of locum cover.

Issues for the patients

- Patient's safety is at risk when a poorly performing GP is allowed to continue to practise.
- Loss of continuity of care while the GP is off sick.

Question 9: Answers

An 80-year-old patient tells you she would like to leave you personally £10,000 in her will.

What do you tell her?

Issues for the patient

- Sign of gratitude for all the years of service by her GP.
- May expect preferential treatment by making this offer (bribe?).
- May be cultural/traditional for the patient's generation and her parents may also have bequeathed a sum to their GP and so on.

Issues for the doctor

- *Probity*: cannot accept for him/herself but may be able to suggest to the patient that she donates the money to her or the practice's favourite charity. Alternatively, if she declines, then you may suggest leaving it to the practice as a whole and not to yourself as an individual.
- Any gift that is not commensurate with the service delivered should be called into question. A bottle of wine at Christmas is acceptable but monetary gifts are more likely to be deemed as a bribe.
- Doctor needs to ascertain whether she is mentally competent to make such a generous gesture. Does she have relatives who would benefit more? Is she under duress?
- Doctor may wish to respect a patient's autonomy and her wish to offer such a generous gift but cannot ethically and morally accept for him/herself.
- Needs to explain to the patient that he/she treats all patients equally and that the NHS is a free medical service for which he/she does not expect any gratuity.
- Needs to be sensitive, as he/she does not want to offend an elderly patient who may have the best intentions by making this gesture.

Issues for the practice

- Any gifts above £100 need to be registered under the Health and Social Care Act Bill (2001) and income tax deducted as appropriate.

- If the sum is accepted by the practice, the practice should use the funds to improve the practice and not distribute the sum as a generous Christmas bonus to all staff.

Wider issues

- Suspicion may be aroused if it becomes public knowledge that a GP has accepted such an amount in a will. This brings into question the probity of the GP and may discredit him/her.
- When is a gift acceptable? What if a drug rep donates £££ to the practice for a practice away day? Or a drug rep pays for an autoclave? This opens up another arena that following the Shipman case and Bristol Infirmary enquiry may fuel mass hysteria about the probity of doctors.

Question 10: Answers

How would you go about setting up a practice protocol for telephone consultations?

- Set *aims* for the telephone consultations. Are they to cut down on emergency consultations? Or to cut down on unnecessary home visits?
- *Background*: what is the evidence that telephone consultations are effective? Is there a gold standard of comparison? NHS Direct has shown that telephone advice for the management of URTIs and low back pain is effective.
- *Target population*: Any registered patient with access to a telephone? But what about refugees, the very young, the infirm, the elderly, the hard of hearing, patients with learning difficulties, disabilities, or language problems? These groups will naturally be excluded. How can they be included?
- *Meeting*: Who needs to be present? Pre-meeting agenda? Arrangement of cover during meeting. Designate chairman. Take minutes.
- *SWOT analysis*: Discuss strengths and weaknesses of telephone consultations, the opportunities to save on home visits and emergency consultations, and the threats—missed diagnosis, inability to perform examination or see patient in person to pick up on cues or red flags, cost, resources (busy phone lines).
- Come up with a *plan* that is realistic, set time, achievable, designate a lead person, devise a timetable or rota of persons manning the phone for consultations.
- *Audit*: Cycle needs to be completed.
- *Management of change*: Set a date of implementation and inform all relevant staff of the telephone protocol. Keep records and reassess after a set time period.
- *Follow-up*: Re-meeting to assess the effectiveness of the telephone consultation protocol and identify areas that need improvement or that have worked effectively.

Question 11: Answers

Comment on the management of the following skin conditions, giving evidence to support your views:

a) **Acne**

Comments	Evidence
Topical preparations for mild-to-moderate acne (benzoyl peroxide, azelaic acid)	*British National Formulary*
Topical antibacterials—erythromycin, clindamycin (may be no more effective than topical benzoyl peroxide and increased resistance to Propionibacterium acnes). This agent is reserved for those who cannot tolerate po	
Topical isotretinoin (acid form of vitamin A) or topical adapalene for mild-to-moderate acne. Side-effects: skin erythema, peeling	
Oral antibiotics (oxytetracycline, tetracycline, doxycycline, minocycline, erythromycin, and trimethoprim) for moderate-to-severe acne. Oxytetracycline or tetracycline 500 mg bd x 3/12. May add a second antibiotic. Expect max results in 6/12 but may need to use for 2 years in severe cases. Co-cyprindiol for women is another option	
Refer to dermatologist for severe acne, acne unresponsive to prolonged courses of oral antibiotics, scarring or associated psychological problems. Patient may be a candidate for oral isotretinoin	

b) **Eczema (allergic, atopic, discoid and venous)**

Comments	Evidence
Removal of skin irritant or contact allergen Emollients (for dry skin, irritant eczema) May supplement with bath or shower emollients	British National Formulary
Topical corticosteroids Mild steroid for face and flexures Potent steroid for discoid or lichenified eczema, scalp, limbs, and trunk Bandages with zinc and ichthammol applied over steroid for limbs for lichenification (from incessant scratching) Topical or systemic antibiotics for secondary infection Refer for severe refractory eczema for phototherapy, systemic steroids or immuno-suppressive agents (ciclosporin, azathioprine or mycophenolate mofetil)	

c) **Psoriasis**

Comments	Evidence
Advised of aggravating factors—lithium, NSAIDs, ACE inhibitors, beta-blockers, chloroquine	British National Formulary
Mild—reassurance and emollient	
UVB phototherapy (mild to moderate, guttate or chronic plaque psoriasis)	
Topical preparations Calcipotriol—plaque psoriasis, scalp, non-staining Coal tar—anti-inflammatory and antiscaling Dithranol—causes skin irritation, apply with care Salicylic acid—descaling Tazarotene—retinoid for mild to moderate	
PUVA (administered in hospital, risk of skin CA)	
Oral retinoids (severe resistant cases). Only prescribed by hospital dermatologist	
Oral immunosuppressants (ciclosporin, methotrexate). Only under supervision of hospital dermatologist.	
Topical or systemic steroids. Only by hospital dermatologist as may precipitate severe pustular psoriasis	

d) **Fungal infections (athlete's foot)**

Comments	Evidence
Allylamines are more effective than placebo	One systemic review and four RCTs in *Clinical Evidence*, June 2004
Azole creams x 4–6/52 increase cure rates *vs* placebo	One RCT in *Clinical Evidence*, June 2004
Advised to avoid swimming pools	One survey showed 9% of swimmers have athlete's foot with the majority being men aged 16 or over. *Clinical Evidence*, 2004

Question 12: Answers

Mrs Fatima Khan, a 34-year-old woman, comes to your surgery and states that she has no interest in sex with her husband. She explains that she has pain during sexual intercourse.

How do you manage this consultation?

Communication issues

- Language barrier? Assess for need of interpreter.
- Cultural barrier? What is her understanding of sexual intercourse?

Issues for the patient

- Relationship with partner. Arranged marriage?
- Depression.
- Embarrassment. She may not reveal much to a male GP. Perhaps a female GP would be better.
- Goaded by partner to see GP? Pressure by partner to have children.

Issues for the doctor

- Non-judgemental approach.
- Take a sensitive history—enquire about the nature of the pain? Is it on initial penetration? Does she feel she is too small and tight to permit penetration? Does she have pain every time she has SI? Does she have a vaginal discharge? Is there foreplay? Is she well lubricated?
- Ask about her relationship with her partner. Is he affectionate? Was the marriage arranged? Does she want children?
- Assess for psychological reasons. Ask about her mood. Is she depressed? What are her views on sex? Has she been raped in the past?
- Perform an abdominal and PV exam.
- Request a health professional chaperone to be present before performing PV exam.
- Discuss the management options with the patient.
- If she has psychological issues causing the vaginismus, consider referring her to a counsellor. Or offer contact details for the British Association for Counselling and Psychotherapy (01788 550899 or access www.counselling.co.uk).

- If she has relationship issues, then encourage her to bring her husband to discuss these or alternatively suggest the practice counsellor or Relate. Contact Relate on 01788 572 241 or access www.relate.org.uk.
- Suggest the penetration desensitisation technique in which she inserts one finger, then two, etc into her vagina while relaxing her muscles.
- If there are deeper psychosexual issues, suggest referring her to a psychosexual therapist at the local FP clinic, Relate or a private therapist through the British Association for Sexual and Relationship Therapy. Provide contact details: 020 8543 2707 or access www.basrt.org.uk.
- Offer self-help books (e.g. Litvinoff S. *The Relate Guide to Sex in Loving Relationships* 2001 or *The Relate Guide to Better Relationships*. London: Vermillion, 1992.)

Evidence-based medicine

- Ryan L, Hawton K. Female dyspareunia. *BMJ* 2004;Jun;328:1357.
- Graziottin A. Clinical approach to dyspareunia. *J Sex Marital Ther* 2001;27:489-501.
- Dean J. ABC of sexual health: examination of patients with sexual problems. *BMJ* 1998;317:Dec:1641–1643.
- Ramage M. ABC of sexual problems: management of sexual problems. *BMJ* 1998 Nov;317:1509–1512.

Written Paper Four

For the Royal College of General Practitioners' Instructions and Glossary for the Written Paper Module, see pages 18–19

Question 1

Olivia, aged 4, is brought to your surgery by her mother. She has a 24-h history of a fever of up to 40 °C.

What do you do?

Question 2

Please read the extract from the paper entitled: Association of deprivation, ethnicity, and sex with quality indicators for diabetes: population based survey of 53,000 patients in primary care (please refer to **Reference material A**), and answer the question given below.

Comment on the strengths and weaknesses of the methodology of subjects for this study.

Reference Material A (Question 2)

Association of deprivation, ethnicity, and sex with quality indicators for diabetes: population based survey of 53,000 patients in primary care.
Hippisley-Cox J, O'Hanlon S, Coupland C.
BMJ *2004* Nov;329:1267–1268.

Methods
The authors identified patients with diabetes over 16 years who were registered with 237 practices included in the new general practice database QRESEARCH (version 3, downloaded on 10 May 2004). This database, which will eventually comprise 500 or more UK general practices, contains Townsend scores derived from the 2001 census (a proxy for material deprivation) and ethnicity, both linked to the output areas associated with each patient's postcode. Output areas consist of about 125 households and are nested within electoral non-white residents in each geographical area. The authors validated the resulting database by comparing against published data on such variables as prevalence of disease, prescriptions, population characteristics, and referral rates, and the authors found similar rates per 1000 population. The authors applied the new general medical services contract queries to the population registered on 1 April 2004 to determine whether each patient was eligible for each target and whether that target had been achieved. Each of the contract targets refer to the care recorded on computer within the past 15 months.

Statistical analysis
The authors derived proportions at practice level and calculated medians and 10th and 90th centiles as a measure of variation between practices. The authors used multilevel logistic regression to determine odds ratios, with 95% confidence intervals, for each indicator comparing patients from the most deprived fifth with those from the most affluent fifth and the fifth of highest ethnicity compared with that of lowest ethnicity, with practice defined as a random effect. The authors also compared men and women. Results were adjusted by age (5-year bands) and sex and deprivation or ethnicity as appropriate. The authors used STATA version 8.2 for all the analyses.

Question 3

Tables from the results section of the paper referred to in question 2 (Association of deprivation, ethnicity, and sex with quality indicators for diabetes: population based survey of 53,000 patients in primary care) are provided (please refer to **Reference material B**).

a) **Interpret the results in the table.**

b) **How might the evidence from the table influence your current practice?**

Reference Material B
(Question 3)

Association of deprivation, ethnicity, and sex with quality indicators for diabetes: population based survey of 53,000 patients in primary care.
Hippisley-Cox J, O'Hanlon S, Coupland C.
BMJ *2004 Nov*;329:1267–1268.

Reproduced with permission from the BMJ Publishing Group.

Table Interpractice variation in percentage of quality indicators for diabetes achieved and associations with deprivation and ethnicity.

Quality indicators	Interpractice variation			Adjusted odds ratio (95% CI)		
	Median	10th centile	90th centile	High deprivation v low (fifths)	High ethnicity v low (fifths)	Women v men
Indicator recorded						
Body mass index	85.8	72.4	93.6	0.86 (0.78–0.95)	0.85 (0.76–0.96)	0.94 (0.9–0.99)
Smoking history	65.2	43.9	83.1	0.68 (0.62–0.74)	1.23 (1.12–1.35)	1.97 (1.90–2.06)
Advice given to smoker	89.5	42.9	100.0	0.96 (0.68–1.37)	1.15 (0.72–1.86)	1.00 (0.83–1.21)
HBA$_{1c}$ concentration	92.2	78.2	97.3	0.82 (0.73–0.93)	0.92 (0.87–1.07)	1.03 (0.97–1.1)
<7.5%	48.0	34.0	62.1	0.88 (0.82–0.95)	0.97 (0.87–1.07)	0.97 (0.93–1.0)
<10%	84.6	69.6	91.8	0.70 (0.64–0.77)	0.83 (0.85–0.92)	1.00 (0.95–1.05)
Blood pressure	95.2	89.4	98.5	0.82 (0.7–0.96)	0.78 (0.66–0.92)	1.15 (1.06–1.25)
<145/85 mm Hg	59.1	43.3	73.1	0.96 (0.9–1.03)	0.96 (0.88–1.04)	0.93 (0.89–0.96)
Creatinine concentration	89.5	76.0	96.3	1.05 (0.94–1.17)	0.79 (0.7–0.89)	0.99 (0.94–1.05)
ACE inhibitors received in presence of proteinuria or microalbuminuria	66.7	0.0	100.0	0.93 (0.68–1.28)	0.77 (0.54–1.0)	0.74 (0.62–0.88)
Serum cholesterol conc	87.0	72.5	95.1	0.93 (0.84–1.02)	0.82 (0.74–0.92)	0.88 (0.83–0.92)
<5 mmol/l	59.8	44.5	74.6	0.99 (0.92–1.06)	0.88 (0.8–0.97)	0.58 (0.56–0.61)
Procedure carried out						
Retinal screening	60.0	25.5	82.7	0.8 (0.74–0.86)	0.94 (0.87–1.03)	0.98 (0.94–1.02)
Pulses checked	53.3	5.7	83.6	0.99 (0.91–1.07)	0.79 (0.7–0.89)	0.94 (0.9–0.99)
Neuropathy test	27.1	0.0	80.4	0.9 (0.81–0.99)	1.17 (1.06–1.29)	0.95 (0.91–1.0)
Microalbuminuria test	39.1	2.7	71.9	0.84 (0.74–0.92)	0.88 (0.79–0.98)	0.91 (0.87–0.96)
Flu vaccination	72.1	57.1	80.9	0.91 (0.84–0.98)	0.76 (0.7–0.83)	0.98 (0.94–1.03)

Question 4

Comment on the management of the following, giving evidence to support your views:

a) **TIA**

Comments	Evidence

b) **Acute stroke**

Comments	Evidence

c) **Secondary prevention of stroke and TIA**

Comments	Evidence

d) Longer-term management of stroke and TIA

Comments	Evidence

Question 5

Joan Walsh, a 50-year-old woman, requests HRT.

How would you manage her?

Question 6

Discuss the issues surrounding appraisal and revalidation of GPs.

Question 7

Mary Lawton is 16 years old and is brought to your surgery by her mother who is concerned that Mary has an eating disorder. Her BMI is 13.

What would you do?

Question 8

You suspect the practice manager of misappropriating funds (£10,000) from the practice.

As her employer, what do you do?

Question 9

Mary Oboku complains of low back pain. Her BMI is 40.

What issues does this raise?

Question 10

Susan Howard, a 45-year-old woman, comes for the results of her thyroid blood test. The test confirms she has hypothyroidism.

How would you manage this consultation?

Question 11

Comment on the following drug side-effects/interactions, citing evidence to support your views:

a) Statins and myopathy

Comments	Evidence

b) Cox-2 inhibitors and cardiovascular risk

Comments	Evidence

c) Depo-provera and bone mineral density

Comments	Evidence

d) Co-proxamol and suicide

Comments	Evidence

Question 12

Mr Richard Lawton, a 66-year-old man, comes to your surgery asking for alternative treatment for his arthritis. He was given rofecoxib based on NICE guidelines, which has now been withdrawn.

How do you manage this consultation?

Question 1: Answers

Olivia, aged 4, is brought to your surgery by her mother. She has a 24-h history of a fever of up to 40 °C.

What do you do?

Communication issues

- Doctor should first speak with the mother to gain the confidence of the child—to appear less of a stranger.
- Doctor should speak in a soft, gentle manner to the child and engage her with light friendly banter, such as "How old are you?", "That's a lovely dress you are wearing", "Do you like Barbie?", "What year are you in at school? Are you in reception?" This should be done prior to any invasive investigations—thermometer or tongue depressor.
- Vary language when wishing to see the back of the throat, "Can I see your back teeth?", as suggested by Neighbours in the Inner Consultation.
- Describe the thermometer as a magic stick or wand as the child will inevitably see the instrument as a syringe for imms.
- Use toys as a nonverbal means of communication.

Issues for the doctor

- Establish rapport with both child and mother to facilitate consultation.
- Provide good clinical care. Full history and examination into the differential diagnoses of high fever—exclude meningitis (rare in general practice), pneumonia, flu or viral rash, gastroenteritis, acute otitis media, UTI, measles, etc. Make sure the child is undressed for a full examination. Check for signs of dehydration—dry tongue, lack of voiding for 8 h or more, tachycardia, etc. Check temperature, TMs for redness or bulging, throat for swollen tonsils or Koplik spots, photophobia, chest for infection, abdomen for loss of bowel sounds, entire skin surface for non-blanching rash, etc.
- Will need a MSU sample if no obvious source is found (in accordance with RCP Guidelines, 1991). 3–5% of girls and 1–2% of boys have UTIs during childhood and, if missed, the consequences may include chronic renal failure with long-term dialysis!
- Self-awareness—having own children allows the doctor to feel comfortable with children, more engaging, and more up-to-date with children's TV

programmes and interests. If the GP is childless, there can be a natural awkwardness in engaging a child.

- Self-awareness of family—are they frequent or rare attenders? Should this matter be given more attention than usual?
- Acknowledge difficulty and possible frustration in examining a febrile, irritable child and the need not to cause further distress.
- Have the child sit on her mother's lap.
- Leave the most distressing part of the examination until last—thermometer and tongue depressor.
- Ensure hands and stethoscope are warm before touching the child's skin.
- Explore mother's anxiety and concerns over child. Has she tried Calpol or ibuprofen? What are her views on medication?

Issues for the mother

- Unable to cope with sick child—reached her limits.
- Unable to sleep at night with sick child.
- Fear of the worst prognosis.
- Loss of control over managing the situation by herself.
- Plea for help. Overworked, domestic stresses? How many children at home?
- Past experience with doctors.

Question 2: Answers

Please read the extract from the paper entitled: Association of deprivation, ethnicity, and sex with quality indicators for diabetes: population based survey of 53,000 patients in primary care (please refer to **Reference material A**) and answer the question given below.

Comment on the strengths and weaknesses of the methodology of subjects for this study.

Strengths

- Cross-sectional survey of 53,000 patients in primary care. Applicable to primary care and not hospital outpatient diabetic clinic.
- Large database of 237 practices.
- Results compared ethnicity, age, sex, and deprivation to avoid confounding variables.
- Sample size is sufficient to detect significant statistical results.
- Odds ratio and 95% confidence intervals calculated.

Weaknesses

- Does not state initial sample size and dropout rate/exclusions with reasons.
- Cross-sectional surveys only provide a snapshot.
- Cannot discuss cause and effect.

Question 3: Answers

Tables from the results section of the paper referred to in question 2 (Association of deprivation, ethnicity, and sex with quality indicators for diabetes: population based survey of 53,000 patients in primary care) are provided (please refer to **Reference material B**).

a) **Interpret the results in the table.**

- 92.2% of patients had their HBA_{1C} measured but only 48% achieved ideal values of <7.5%.
- Serum cholesterol and BMI were recorded in most practices.
- Microalbuminuria and neuropathy were poorly recorded: 39.1% and 27.1%, respectively.
- Patients from areas of high deprivation were less likely to have records of BMI, smoking status, BP, HBA_{1C} concentration, retinal screening, neuropathy testing, microalbuminuria testing, or flu vaccination.
- Patients from areas of high ethnicity were less likely to have records of BMI, BP, pulses, creatinine concentration, cholesterol concentration, an HBA_{1C} of <10%, microalbuminuia testing, or flu vaccination.
- Patients from areas of high ethnicity were more likely to have records of neurological testing and smoking history.
- Women were less likely to have records of BMI, pulses, BP <145/85 mm Hg, microalbuminuria testing, serum cholesterol concentration, or treatment with ACEI in the presence of microalbuminuria or proteinuria.
- Women were more likely to have smoking and BP records. However, these checks are used for oral contraceptives and HRT, which are confounding factors.

b) **How might the evidence from the table influence your current practice?**

- As I work in a high deprivation area with high ethnicity, this highlights the need to improve diabetic reviews in my practice patients. Perhaps an additional session with a diabetic specialist nurse may need to be implemented to provide adequate diabetic reviews to these population groups.
- It highlights the need for practices in areas of high deprivation and high ethnicity to provide better access to their diabetic patients and a more thorough review. Perhaps instigate a method to chase up diabetic patients and invite them for reviews. Target ethnic groups by having an ethnic diabetic nurse.

Question 4: Answers

Comment on the management of the following, giving evidence to support your views:

a) **TIA**

Comments	Evidence
Patients with >1 TIA in a week should be referred to hospital immediately for investigation Once symptoms have resolved, aspirin 300 mg od should be initiated Patients who have made a good recovery should be assessed and investigated in a neurovascular clinic within 7 days	The Intercollegiate Working Party for Stroke. *Royal College of Physicians National Clinical Guidelines for Stroke*, 2nd edn. London: RCP, 2004
Antiplatelet therapy reduces the risk of serious vascular event in patients with prior TIA or stroke Antihypertensive therapy reduces stroke in people with prior TIA or stroke	*Clinical Evidence,* 2004

b) **Acute stroke**

Comments	Evidence
Admit and manage on a stroke unit with access to specialist palliative care. Brain imaging within 24 h of onset and urgently if the patient is on anticoagulants, has a depressed LOC, has a known bleeding tendency, has fever, neck stiffness or papilloedema, has severe headache at onset, has unexplained fluctuating symptoms, or has indication for thrombolysis or early anticoagulation. If not admitted to hospital, patients should be managed by a specialist stroke rehab team	The Intercollegiate Working Party for Stroke. *Royal College of Physicians National Clinical Guidelines for Stroke*, 2nd edn. London: RCP, 2004
Aspirin within 48 h of ischaemic stroke confirmed by CT, reduces death or dependency at 6 months and increases complete recovery *vs* placebo	*Clinical Evidence* 2004

Comments	Evidence
Specialist stroke rehab reduces death and dependency after a median follow-up of 1 year	*Clinical Evidence* 2004
Thrombolysis reduces risk of death and dependency after 1–6 months but increases death from intracranial bleed in the first 7–10 days and after 1–6 months. Acute reduction of BP may have a worse clinical outcome and increased mortality	*Clinical Evidence* 2004

c) **Secondary prevention of stroke and TIA**

Comments	Evidence
One stroke increases risk of further stroke by 30–43% within 5 years and is highest early after stroke or TIA Advice on lifestyle: stop smoking, diet, weight, reduce salt, avoid excess alcohol, regular exercise Inclusion on stroke register and annual follow-up Annual flu vaccination Treat high BP that persists for 2 weeks	The Intercollegiate Working Party for Stroke. *Royal College of Physicians National Clinical Guidelines for Stroke*, 2nd edn. London: RCP, 2004
Aim for a BP <140/<85 mm Hg Recommend thiazide (bendroflumethiazide or indapamide) or an ACEI (perindopril or ramipril) or both unless C/I Start 75 mg aspirin or 75 mg clopidogrel or combo of aspirin and dipyridamole MR 200 mg bd if not on anticoagulation after TIA or ischaemic stroke Anticoagulaton should be started in patients with atrial fibrillation Anticoagulation should be started after CT scan has excluded haemorrhage and not until 14 days have passed from onset of an ischaemic stroke Start statin (40 mg simvastatin) in patients with ischaemic stroke or TIA + TC >3.5 mmol/L unless C/I	BHS-IV guidelines

d) **Longer-term management of stroke and TIA**

Comments	Evidence
Access to specialist care and rehab Encourage independence Address the needs of the carers (high morbidity) Ensure access to information about statutory and voluntary organisations GPs should keep a register of stroke patients and conduct a regular audit of secondary prevention and management of chronic disability By 6 months, over half will still need assistance with activities of daily living. 15% have communication impairment and 53% have motor weakness	The Intercollegiate Working Party for Stroke. *Royal College of Physicians Clinical Guidelines for Stroke*, 2nd edn. London: RSM, 2004 New GMS Contract

Question 5: Answers

Joan Walsh, a 50-year-old woman, requests HRT.

How would you manage her?

Issues for the patient

- What are her ideas about HRT? Concerns about her health and expectations from the drug? Is it for distressing menopausal symptoms or does she falsely believe that it is cardioprotective or that it will prevent osteoporosis?

Issues for the doctor

- Confirm menopause—FSH level >30 + symptoms.
- Self-awareness—the use of HRT by women aged 50–64 in the UK over the past 10 years has resulted in an estimated 20,000 additional breast cancers. The *Lancet* in 2002 reported that the use of HRT over a 5-year period was estimated to cause about 6 extra cases of breast cancer per 1000 users between ages 50 and 55, and 12 per 1000 aged 60–69; the figure was raised to 19 per 1000 women on HRT in the UK 'Million Women Study' (UK 'Million Women Study' Collaborators. Breast cancer and hormone-replacement therapy in the Million Women Study. *Lancet* 2003;363:419–427).
- Inform patient of the risks of HRT (increased risk of breast cancer in long-term users, venous thrombosis, stroke, and ovarian cancer in hysterectomised women on oestrogen-only HRT). Need to warn the patient about HRT causing breast cancer or face litigation after mass media hype. The relative risk is 1.66 for incidence of breast cancer and 1.22 for death from breast cancer. Use layman's terms.
- If she wants HRT for osteoporosis prevention, suggest other options, such as selective oestrogen receptor modulators, bisphosphonates (an effective, nonhormonal treatment), calcium, and vitamin D compounds. The Royal College of Physicians Guidelines on the treatment of osteoporosis endorse bisphosphonates for fracture protection.
- Inform patient of the potential side-effects of HRT: heavy periods, tender breasts, weight gain.
- Inform patient of the benefits of short-term use of HRT for 2–3 years as recommended by the Committee on Safety of Medicines—relief of menopausal symptoms of hot flushes and night sweats. Explain to her that

hot flushes tend to peak in the first year after periods stop (the climacteric) and usually settle within 2–5 years. Explain that 80% of women suffer hot flushes during the menopause but that only 20% feel the symptoms warrant medical attention. Other benefits include reducing vaginal dryness and questionable benefit of relieving mood swings and depression.

- Discuss alternative medication for hot flushes—clonidine (35% effective), fluoxetine (50%), megestrol acetate (85%), paroxetine (65%), progesterone (83%), and venlafaxine (50–60%).
- Give patient all the evidence to make an informed decision.
- Review patient at least annually while on HRT to discuss risk:benefit for continuing treatment.

Evidence-based medicine

- Women's Health Initiative (WHI) study on HRT, July 2002, was stopped early as taking combined HRT for >5 years was clearly shown to increase risks of breast cancer and venous thromboembolic disease. Also, the risk of heart attack and stroke was increased over 1 year by 7 in 10,000 and 8 in 10,000, respectively.
- Beral V, Banks E, Reeves G. Evidence from randomised trials on the long-term effects of HRT. *Lancet* 2002;Sep;360:942–944.
- UK 'Million Women Study' Collaborators. Breast cancer and hormone-replacement therapy in the Million Women Study. *Lancet* 2003;363:419–427.
  — Confirmed that there is a small increase in risk of breast cancer in association with oestrogen-only products (taking oestrogen-only HRT for 10 years increases breast cancer risk by about 5 in 1000 or 0.5% over 10 years).
  — There is a substantially greater increase in risk of breast cancer in association with the use of combined oestrogen and progesterone HRT than with oestrogen-only therapy. Study showed that taking combined HRT for 5 and 10 years increases risk of breast cancer by 6 in 1000 women (0.6% over 5 years) and 19 in 1000 women (1.9% over 10 years), respectively.
  — Breast cancer mortality was increased (relative risk 1.22) in women on HRT.
  — Background risk of developing breast cancer in postmenopausal women is 2%, which is doubled by taking combined HRT.
- Committee on Safety of Medicines
  — Long-term HRT does not reduce coronary heart disease in women and may increase its incidence slightly in early use.
  — There is an increase in risk of stroke in HRT users.
  — Baseline risk of VTE in non-HRT users aged between 50 and 70 is higher than previously estimated so the absolute risk associated with HRT is also higher.
  — HRT should only be prescribed for the short-term relief of menopausal symptoms and prevention of osteoporosis.

Question 6: Answers

Discuss the issues surrounding appraisal and revalidation of GPs.

Issues for the patients

- Fuelled by media attention to Dr Shipman, the Bristol Infirmary enquiry, etc, in an attempt to ensure all GPs are safe.
- Even patient satisfaction surveys are not entirely valid to measure a GP's fitness to practise. According to the 360° feedback study, patients were more concerned with being heard and being told what would happen by their GP than with a GP's clinical competence, actions in emergency situations, and maintaining confidentiality (areas that colleagues and doctors found important).

Issues for the GP

- Appraisal and revalidation are tools devised by the GMC and implemented by the respective PCTs to check a doctor's fitness to practise.
- The GMC now insists on annual appraisals and 5-yearly revalidation for doctors to remain registered with it in order to, "safeguard the highest standards of medical ethics, education, and practice in the interest of patients, the public, and the profession."
- Professor Sir Graeme Catto, President of the GMC, implemented reforms of medical regulation on 1 November 2004; these addressed a doctor's fitness to practise in the round, and introduced division of investigation and adjudication, warnings, and a new single test when doctors are referred for investigation.
- Appraisal is based on the seven codes of Good Medical Practice: providing good clinical care, maintaining good medical practice, working with colleagues, teaching and assessing, respecting patients, probity, and own health.
- Need for impartial process, appraisal by a doctor outside of own practice, preferably another GP. A doctor cannot fail an appraisal.
- Is self-regulation by appraisal a valid process? Would Dr Shipman have passed scrutiny by being appraised annually? Is this truly a valid instrument to assess a doctor's fitness to practise and identify poorly performing doctors? A GP can also achieve quality markers if well organised. Is the use of indicators to measure clinical governance performance any better? What about other quality markers such as MAP, MRCGP, quality practice awards, FRCGP? What value will be placed on this?

- Positive aspect of appraisal—formulating own personal development plan, encouraging self-regulation, learning tool.

Issues for the NHS

- Cost issue for the PCT—pays £400 to each GP who is appraised by an appointed appraiser from the PCT. The appraiser will also need to be reimbursed for his/her time.
- Criteria to be appraiser? Who decides on these criteria?
- Resources—time and expense for PCT to appraise all GPs (partners, salaried and locum).
- Consequences for doctors who do poorly on appraisals and revalidation? Resources to retrain GPs? Who will pay? There is already a shortage of GPs. Will single-handed GPs be treated differently—singled out by the PCT in an attempt to retire them all to avoid another Shipman? Is this another tool for the PCT to exert more influence over GPs?

Issues for the government

- Does it stop with appraisal, revalidation, clinical governance, new GMC test of Fitness to Practise, or will the government be persuaded by media and public pressure to introduce GP league tables, register of visits by drug reps, etc? When will the policing of GPs stop? When will the public be satisfied that Dr Shipman was a one-off psychopath and leave GPs to do what they do best—practise medicine? Why are GPs being singled out?
- Fundamental issue is 'when will government/public involvement and scrutiny back down?' or is it inevitable that GPs will become obsolete? More GPs turn to freelance work and part-time posts, rather than taking up partnership. Others take early retirement in an attempt to avoid more paperwork and government interference. General practice is no longer about being a good GP but rather conducting audits, IT, receiving PACT data, referral patterns, etc. Would medical students become GPs if they knew the level of government policing they would face?

Evidence-based medicine

- McDermott A, Hasler J. 360° feedback: how do perceptions of doctors' attributes compare? *Clin Gov Bull* 2004;5(4). Study analysed the views of almost 4000 patients and 3000 colleagues on doctors' performance and found that doctors are less positive about themselves than are their patients and colleagues.
- General Medical Council. *Good Medical Practice*, 3rd edn. London: GMC, 2001. www.gmc-uk.org

- Chambers R, Wakley G, Field S, Ellis S. *Appraisal for the Apprehensive* 2002: *a Guide for Doctors*. Oxford: Radcliffe Medical Press.
- Conlon M. Appraisal: the catalyst of personal development. *BMJ* 2003;327:389–391.
- www.doh.gov.uk/ gpappraisal/
- www.appraisals.nhs.uk/
- www.revalidationuk.info/
- www.gmc-uk.org/revalidation

Question 7: Answers

Mary Lawton is 16 years old and is brought to your surgery by her mother who is concerned that Mary has an eating disorder. Her BMI is 13.

What would you do?

Issues for the patient

- Respect patient's autonomy. She may refuse intervention. She may be in denial. Does she want to be seen alone?
- Check patient's understanding of her condition and of her mother's concern. "Do you think you have an eating problem?"
- Determine her ideas about her body image, concerns about being too fat, and expectations from the doctor or from her family.
- Is this a coping strategy for abuse at home? Why does she feel she has no control in her life except over her body?

Issues for the doctor

- Provide good clinical care. A BMI of <17.5 kg/m^2 is diagnostic. Look for signs of anorexia—lanugo hair, amenorrhoea, distorted body image, blackouts, over-activity, bradycardia, hypotension, cold cyanotic extremities, and muscle atrophy.
- If bulimic, check for dental caries, enlarged salivary glands, and petechiae on the sclera. Other signs are hypokalaemia and menstrual irregularities.
- Useful investigations—FBC (anaemia, leucopaenia, thrombocytopaenia), urea and electrolytes (renal failure), glucose, calcium, phosphate, LFTs, and serum proteins. Additional tests include ECG (bradycardia, arrhythmias, and conduction defects) and a bone density scan (osteoporosis).
- Look for concurrent psychiatric morbidity—personality disorders, major depression, OCD, anxiety or substance misuse.
- Self-awareness—doctor realises that he/she may need to use the Mental Health Act and arrange emergency hospital admission if he/she believes the patient's life is in serious danger from the illness. He/she may need to enlist the support of the mother. Address patient's denial and resistance.
- Multidisciplinary team approach—Mary needs psychological therapy (CBT, focused psychodynamic therapy or motivation enhancement), nutritional rehabilitation, and management of her physical ailments.

189

- Aware that an eating disorder in an adolescent may be a sign of being a victim of abuse. Arrange family therapy and ascertain family dynamics.
- Aware that 43% recover and 36% improve, but 5% die from suicide or cardiac complications.
- Self-awareness—doctor may feel emotionally upset by seeing an emaciated adolescent, and may have children of his/her own; may need to do some housekeeping before seeing the next patient.

Evidence-based medicine

- www.nice.org.uk/pdf/cg009quickrefguide.pdf.
- www.edauk.com (UK charity aimed at young people with eating disorders).

Question 8: Answers

You suspect the practice manager of misappropriating funds (£10,000) from the practice.

As her employer, what do you do?

Medicolegal issues

- Gather evidence and contact your antifraud officer for the PCT.
- Do not confront the practice manager as she may destroy the evidence.
- National fraud and corruption reporting line for the NHS: 08702 400 100.
- NHS Counter Fraud and Security Management Service in London: 020 7895 4500.

Issues for the practice manager (employee)

- Is she under personal or family stress or financial burden?
- Is she misusing substances?
- Is she unwell?
- Perhaps she has no insight?

Issues for the GP (employer)

- Gather evidence—access the records, invoices, and bank statements of the practice. Any witnesses? Notify the antifraud officer for the PCT.
- Self-awareness—need to be sensitive. Personal conflict between feelings and duty as the practice manager may be well liked.
- GP should meet with the other partners and discuss the matter with concrete evidence at hand. Options here are for mandatory dismissal or to show leniency. One partner may argue that if she can repay the practice, if the reason is exceptional, if she shows remorse, the partners should show compassion due to length of service and circumstances. However, this is not possible as employer–employee trust has been breached by the practice manager and she has committed a criminal offence (fraud and theft).
- Acknowledge that as an employer running a business you must comply with employment laws when addressing circumstances that lead to dismissal. As from 1 October 2004, employers and employees have been

required by law to try to resolve problems before they escalate and end up in an Employment Tribunal—Employment Act (2002) (Dispute Resolution) Regulations (2004).

- *Procedure*:
  - — Step 1: written notification if the partners decide that she must be dismissed. GP should provide the practice manager with written information of grievances that have led to dismissal for gross misconduct. In cases of less serious grievances, an invitation to attend a practice meeting to discuss the problem is extended.
  - — Step 2: Practice meeting for less serious grievances. The employee has a right to be accompanied to this 'hearing'. The main objective of the practice meeting is to try to resolve the problem. All parties concerned will be able to discuss their views in a non-judgemental atmosphere with an appointed chairman (senior partner) and minutes should be recorded. The GP can only make a decision as to how to proceed with the complaint against the employee after the meeting and not during. After the meeting, the employer should inform the employee of the decision and also of her right to appeal. In this situation of gross misconduct, step 2 is omitted.
  - — Step 3: If requested, an appeal meeting is held and chaired by a more senior person (request a member of the LMC or BMA). The appeal decision is then communicated to the employee.
- *Probity:* In this particular matter, the police will need to be notified, as the practice manager is accused of fraud. Contact the police only after conclusive evidence is established and do not base your decision on circumstantial evidence.
- GP may need to read up on employment law and antifraud guidance.

Issues for the practice

- Loss of funds impacts on the practice's resources.
- Chaos, as the practice will need to employ a new practice manager.
- Uneasy atmosphere among employees.
- Institute an antifraud policy—two doctors' signatures on cheques, reconcile invoices and bank statements frequently, division of labour (ordering *vs* invoicing), cheques for signing should be attached to the invoice, receipts for all petty cash transactions, etc.
- The Chartered Institute of Management Accountants publishes an advice sheet on which situations can lead to fraud: poor staff relations, no employee screening, staff redundancies, personal financial pressures, poor wages, employees working antisocial hours without supervision. Suspicion should be raised if records have been altered, e.g. use of tippex, photocopies of bank statements or invoices (not original), lifestyle discrepancy with pay, supplies exceeding need, unexplained fluctuations in account balances.
- Counter-fraud measures saved the NHS £478 million in 2003–4.

Question 9: Answers

Mary Oboku complains of low back pain. Her BMI is 40.

What issues does this raise?

Issues for the patient

- Embarrassment or denial about weight?
- Low self-esteem resulting in overeating.
- Cultural acceptance of being obese and may even be deemed as desirable in Afro-Caribbean women.
- Reached her back pain threshold and so has come to the GP.
- Ideas about what is causing her back pain. Does she have insight?
- What does she expect from her GP?

Issues for the doctor

- Management of obesity in the patient whose BMI is >30.
- Management of low back pain—exclude yellow and red flags. Offer simple analgesia and advice on back strengthening exercises.
- Patient-centred approach to the consultation as patient must be ready to diet and take up exercise.
- Self-awareness that many patients do not take their doctor's advice to lose weight and exercise. Patients often state that they eat hardly anything and don't understand why they are overweight.
- Self-awareness that the GP may find obese patients repulsive and consider them lazy; reaffirmation of society's prejudice.
- Mary is at higher risk of coronary heart disease, gallstones, ovarian cancer, osteoarthritis, sleep apnoea, dyslipidaemia, etc. Doctor needs to exclude these medical conditions and make the patient aware of these added health risks.
- Involve patient's family to offer support and encouragement to Mary.
- Suggest a food diary.
- Arrange blood tests for FBG and fasting cholesterol. Calculate her 10-year coronary heart disease risk.
- Exclude medical causes of obesity, such as hypothyroidism, diabetes, PCO, Cushing's syndrome, use of steroids.
- Obese patients often have raised blood pressures. Monitor Mary's BP.
- Refer to hospital dietician.

- National Institute of Health has issued guidelines on management of obesity. Offer drug treatment—orlistat for obese adults whose BMI is ≥30. May discuss with Mary that if she can lose 2.5 kg she is eligible for this weight-reducing pill.
- Encourage lifestyle changes—change of diet and taking up exercise.

Issues for the practice

- Need to purchase thigh-sized BP cuffs for obese patients.
- Need to purchase weighing scales to accommodate the very obese.
- Need to ensure seats in the waiting room and consulting rooms are sturdy enough to support the weight of obese patients.
- Need to offer a non-judgemental atmosphere to obese patients.

Question 10: Answers

Susan Howard, a 45-year-old woman, comes for the results of her thyroid blood test. The test confirms she has hypothyroidism.

How would you manage this consultation?

Issues for the patient

- Uncertainty, lack of knowledge regarding the condition.
- Fear and anxiety over a chronic condition, its prognosis, and treatment.

Issues for the doctor

- Need to show sensitivity and explore her ideas, concerns, and expectations with respect to thyroid disease. Educate her.
- Need to address her psychological needs—fears, anxieties.
- Need to establish whether she has autoimmune thyroiditis, subacute thyroiditis, or Hashimoto's thyroiditis.
- Arrange further blood tests—autoantibodies, antithyroglobulin, and antiperoxidase, fasting lipids, fasting glucose, and HbA_{1C}. Primary hypothyroidism may be associated with diabetes, hypercholesterolaemia, or pernicious anaemia.
- Need to exclude drug causes of thyroid disease. Is she on amiodarone, lithium, interferon alpha, interleukin 2, iodine, etc?
- Examine her for bradycardia, carpal tunnel syndrome, proximal weakness, goitre, Pemberton's sign, peripheral neuropathy, and vitiligo.
- Examine her eyes for proptosis, periorbital oedema, restrictive extraocular myopathy, etc.
- Starting dose is 50–100 µg of thyroxine od. If there is concomitant heart disease, reduce to 25 µg. Warn patient of potential side-effects of diarrhoea, insomnia, restlessness, angina pain if dose is too high.
- Monitor TFTs. Changes in TSH concentration take 4–6 weeks.
- Provide information on access to a specialist endocrine nurse or self-help group.
- Inform the patient she is entitled to free prescriptions and complete a prescription charge exemption certificate.
- Refer to endocrine specialist if she has ischaemic heart disease, is pregnant or postpartum, has evidence of pituitary disease, or is on amiodarone or lithium therapy.

Issues for the practice

- Audit registered patients with thyroid disease. Are they being reviewed regularly? Medication reviews? TFT monitoring?

Evidence

- Lindsay RS, Toft AD. Hypothyroidism. *Lancet* 1997 Feb;349:413–416.
- Rehman HU, Bajwa TA. Newly diagnosed hypothyroidism. *BMJ* 2004 Nov;329:1271.

Question 11: Answers

Comment on the following drug side-effects/interactions citing evidence to support your views:

a) **Statins and myopathy**

Comments	Evidence
OTC simvastatin 10 mg—LFTs not required	British Heart Foundation, 2004
Higher doses require LFTs within 1–3 months, then every 6 months for 1 year	
Simvastatin and atorvastatin are metabolised by cytochrome P450. The risk of myopathy is increased with amiodarone, diazepam, and verapamil (less potent inhibitors of CYP3A4), and also by 'azole' antifungals or HIV-protease inhibitors	Committee on Safety of Medicines, Oct 2004
Grapefruit juice should be avoided as this can increase exposure to simvastatin	

b) **Cox-2 inhibitors and cardiovascular risk**

Comments	Evidence
Rofecoxib (Vioxx) was withdrawn by its manufacturers, MSD. Data showed that use of Vioxx for 9 months increased risk of MI or CVA. Risk is one event in every 125 years of patient treatment	US Food and Drug Administration
No significant difference in CV events between diclofenac 50 mg and etoricoxib 90 mg for 1 yr	MSD's EDGE randomised trial with 7111 patients. Am College of Rheum meeting
Valdecoxib (Bextra) increases risk of CV event post CABG surgery	Pfizer's two studies of 1500 patients

c) **Depo-provera and bone mineral density**

Comments	Evidence
Depo-provera should only be prescribed in adolescents as first-line if all other methods have been discussed and are deemed unacceptable as depo is associated with bone mineral density reduction	Committee on Safety of Medicine
Use of depo should be discussed every 2 years	

d) **Co-proxamol and suicide**

Comments	Evidence
Co-proxamol contains 32.5 mg of dextropro-poxyphene and 325 mg of paracetamol. It is the former constituent that causes fatal arrhythmias and apnoea. Between 300 and 400 people die each year in England and Wales from co-proxamol OD. MHRA announced phased withdrawal of co-proxamol in January 2005 following assessment of its risks vs benefits	Committee on Safety of Medicines, 2005 www.mhra.gov.uk
Of 4162 drug-related suicides 1997–99, 18% (766) involved co-proxamol alone, highest in the 10–24 age group. Odds of dying after overdose were 2.3 times that of TCAs and 28.1 times that of paracetamol	Hawton K et al, BMJ 2003;326:1006 Co-proxamol and suicide: a study of national mortality and statistics of local non-fatal self poisonings
Advises reduction of access to means of suicide	National Institute for Mental Health in England: Preventing Suicide (national suicide prevention strategy)

Question 12: Answers

Mr Richard Lawton, a 66-year-old man, comes to your surgery, asking for alternative treatment for his arthritis. He was given rofecoxib based on NICE guidelines, which has now been withdrawn.

How do you manage this consultation?

Issues for the patient

- Pain control of his arthritis.
- Maintaining an active lifestyle.
- Concern regarding the effects of rofecoxib and his risk of stroke or MI.
- Seeking information and reassurance.

Issues for the doctor

- Withdrawal of this selective Cox-2 inhibitor has opened the doors to many arthritic patients consulting their GP for reassurance and alternative medication.
- Less choice of gastroprotective anti-inflammatory drugs for doctor to manage arthritis.
- Assess Mr Lawton's risk of cardiovascular disease. Reassure him that he has not caused damage thus far by taking rofecoxib.
- Rofecoxib and etoricoxib (Arcoxia) are both sulphones. How safe then is etoricoxib?
- Celecoxib (Celebrex) and valdecoxib (Bextra) are sulphonamides. Is it safer then to prescribe these Cox-2 inhibitors instead?
- Lumiracoxib (Prexige) is a newer Cox-2 inhibitor structurally related to diclofenac. Not yet released so too new to decide.
- Options for the management of Mr Lawton's arthritis if he has no risk factor for cardiovascular disease include commencing a low dose of celecoxib or valdecoxib.
- Options for the management of Mr Lawton's arthritis if he is at risk of CV disease include partially selective Cox-2 inhibitors which are less effective at reducing GI side-effects but are also less likely to cause CV events. The choices are meloxicam, etodolac, and aceclofenac.
- Another option is to reassess the need for NSAIDs. If required, then perhaps offer ibuprofen, diclofenac, ketoprofen, naproxen, or piroxicam and add a proton-pump inhibitor, H_2 blocker or misoprostol. The dilemma is

that Mr Lawton is over 65 and is therefore at added risk of developing a serious GI adverse event. According to a recent article in the *BMJ* (see below), misoprostol + Cox-2 or selective NSAIDs reduces the risk of symptomatic ulcers and serious GI complications.

- Offer more frequent follow-up to monitor for GI adverse side-effects, BP, and renal function.

Evidence-based medicine

- Vioxx (rofecoxib) was withdrawn by the manufacturers following discussions with the US Food and Drug Administration. Data showed that patients who took Vioxx for >9 months were at increased risk of MI or stroke. The risk was calculated to be one event in every 125 years of patient treatment.
- Hooper L, Brown TJ, Elliott RA, *et al.* The effectiveness of five strategies for the prevention of gastrointestinal toxicity induced by non-steroidal anti-inflammatory drugs: systematic review. *BMJ* 2004 Oct;329:948–952.

Written Paper Five

For the Royal College of General Practitioners' Instructions and Glossary for the Written Paper Module, see pages 18–19

Question 1

Mark Simons, a 15-year old, is brought in by his parents as he is suffering from depression. The mother asks you to prescribe Prozac.

Discuss your management.

Question 2

Please read the extract from the paper entitled: The effectiveness of five strategies for the prevention of gastrointestinal toxicity induced by non-steroidal anti-inflammatory drugs: systematic review (please refer to **Reference material A**), and answer the question given below.

Comment on the strengths and weaknesses of the methodology of study population for this study.

Reference Material A
(Question 2)

The effectiveness of five strategies for the prevention of gastrointestinal toxicity induced by non-steroidal anti-inflammatory drugs: systematic review.
Hooper L, Brown TJ, Elliott RA, *et al.*
BMJ 2004 Oct;329:948–950.

Methods

Searching
The authors searched the Cochrane Library, Medline, Embase, Current Controlled Trials, and System for Information on Grey Literature in Europe (SIGLE) in May 2002.

Selection
The authors rejected articles only if the reviewers could determine that the article was not a randomised controlled trial; the trial did not address any of the five treatment strategies compared with non-selective NSAIDs alone; the trial included exclusively children or healthy volunteers; the study period was less than 21 days, or none of our outcomes were measured.

Primary outcomes were serious gastrointestinal complications (including haemorrhage, haemorrhagic erosions, recurrent upper GI bleeds, perforation, pyloric obstruction, melaena); symptomatic ulcers; serious cardiovascular or renal illness; health-related quality of life (not measures of arthritis pain or disability); and mortality.

Secondary outcomes included total gastrointestinal symptoms, endoscopic ulcers, anaemia, occult bleeding, total dropouts, and dropouts owing to gastrointestinal symptoms.

Validity assessment
Quality assessment of randomised controlled trials included information on randomisation procedures, allocation concealment, similarity at baseline, blinding of participants, providers of care and assessors of outcomes, and losses to follow-up. The authors based the summary risk of bias on assessment of allocation concealment and baseline comparability.

Quantitative data synthesis
Where appropriate the reviewers used relative risks in random effects meta-analysis. The reviewers performed random effects meta-regression to analyse associations between treatment effect and duration of follow-up; participants' mean age; baseline gastrointestinal status (quantified as percentage of participants with a history of ulcers or bleeds); and number of initial risk factors for gastrointestinal toxicity. The outcome was symptomatic ulcers.

Question 3

Forrest plot Tables from the results section of the paper referred to in question 2 (The effectiveness of five strategies for the prevention of gastrointestinal toxicity induced by non-steroidal anti-inflammatory drugs: systematic review) are provided (please refer to **Reference material B**).

Interpret the results in Table 3.

Reference Material B (Question 3)

The effectiveness of five strategies for the prevention of gastrointestinal toxicity induced by non-steroidal anti-inflammatory drugs: systematic review.
Hooper L, Brown TJ, Elliott RA, *et al.*
BMJ 2004 Oct;329:948–950.

Table 3 Effects of gastroprotective strategies on serious gastrointestinal complications.

Study or subcategory	Gastroprotector n/N	Placebo n/N	Relative risk 95% CI	Weight	Relative risk 95% CI
Proton pump inhibitors v placebo					
Ekstrom 1996	0/85	0/90			Not estimable
Blancho Porro 1998	0/50	1/53		33.57	0.35 (0.01–8.47)
Hawkey 1998b	0/274	1/155		33.21	0.19 (0.01–4.61)
Graham 2002	1/268	0/133		33.22	1.49 (0.06–36.44)
Subtotal (95% CI)	677	431		100.00	0.46 (0.07–2.92)
Test for heterogeneity: X^2= 0.85, df=2, P=0.65					
Test for overall effect: z=0.82, P=0.41					
Misoprostol v placebo					
Graham 1998	1/283	0/138		2.17	1.47 (0.06–35.81)
Bolton 1989	0/31	1/36		2.21	0.39 (0.02–9.13)
Chandrasekaran 1991	0/45	0/45			Not estimable
Doherty 1992	0/228	0/227			Not estimable
Melo Gomes 1993	0/216	5/427		2.65	0.18 (0.01–3.23)
Delmas 1994	0/102	0/84			Not estimable
Eliot 1994	0/40	0/43			Not estimable
Silverstein 1995	25/4404	42/4439		90.82	0.6(0.37–0.98)
Hawkey 1998b	0/297	1/155		2.17	0.17 (0.01–4.26)
Graham 2002	0/134	0/133			Not estimable
Subtotal (95% CI)	5780	5727		100.00	0.57 (0.36–0.91)
Total events: 26 (gastroprotector), 49 (placebo)					
Test for heterogeneity: X^2= 1.59, df=4, P=0.81					
Test for overall effect: z=2.33, P=0.02					

0.01　0.1　1　10　100
Favours gastroprotector　Favours placebo

Table 3 – *continued*

Study or subcategory	Gastroprotector n/N	Placebo n/N	Relative risk 95% CI	Weight	Relative risk 95% CI
Specific Cox-2 v Cox-1					
Benson 1999	0/399	1/198		1.38	0.17 (0.01–4.05)
Emery 1999	0/326	1/329		1.38	0.34 (0.01–8.23)
Laine 1999	1/381	2/183		2.46	0.24 (0.02–2.63)
Simon 1999	0/693	1/225		1.38	0.11 (0.00–2.66)
Bombardier 2000	18/4047	39/4029		45.4	0.46 (0.26–0.8)
CLASS 2000	20/3987	24/3981		40.19	0.83 (0.46–1.5)
Cannon 2000	0/516	0/268			Not estimable
Hawkey 2000	0/369	1/187		1.38	0.17 (0.01–4.14)
Dougados 2001	0/80	1/90		1.39	0.37 (0.02–9.06)
Goldstein 2001	2/269	2/270		3.69	1.00 (0.14–7.07)
Kivitz 2001	0/420	1/207		1.38	0.16 (0.01–4.03)
Subtotal (95% CI)	11 487	9967		100.00	0.55 (0.38–0.80)

Test for heterogeneity: X²= 5.86, df=9, P=0.75
Test for overall effect: z=3.11, P=0.002

Favours gastroprotector — Favours placebo

210

Question 4

Discuss the usefulness of the following drugs in the treatment of heart failure, giving evidence to support your views:

a) ACE inhibitors

Comments	Evidence

b) Beta-blockers

Comments	Evidence

c) Digoxin

Comments	Evidence

d)   **Angiotensin II receptor blockers**

Comments	Evidence

Question 5

Mrs Barry brings in her 4-year-old son, who is small for his age. He has a history of frequent chest infections and bulky, greasy stools. You suspect cystic fibrosis.

How would you manage this patient?

Question 6

Mrs Keegan brings in her 7-year-old son, Matthew, to your surgery. She reports that he wets the bed every night.

How would you manage this consultation?

Question 7

Discuss the usefulness of the following interventions for smoking cessation, giving evidence to support your views:

a) Advice on smoking cessation

Comments	Evidence

b) Bupropion for smoking cessation

Comments	Evidence

c) Nicotine replacement therapy for smoking cessation

Comments	Evidence

Question 8

Discuss how you would develop a practice protocol for diabetic care.

Question 9

Mr Santos holds you hostage in your room. He demands a sick note from you for his probation officer and tells you that he will go to jail if you do not issue one. He raises his voice and stands above you menacingly.

What do you do? What issues does this raise?

Question 10

Discuss the usefulness of the following interventions for secondary prevention of ischaemic heart events, citing evidence to support your views:

a) Advice on lifestyle

Comments	Evidence

b) Aspirin

Comments	Evidence

c) Beta-blockers

Comments	Evidence

d) **ACE inhibitors**

Comments	Evidence

Question 11

Mrs Charlotte Winter brings in her baby, Louisa, to your surgery. She states that she thinks her baby is allergic to peanuts.

What do you do?

Question 12

Comment on the following, citing evidence to support your views:

a) Benefit of patient-centred consultations

Comments	Evidence

b) Heartsink patients and communication skills

Comments	Evidence

Question 1: Answers

Mark Simons, a 15-year old, is brought in by his parents as he is suffering from depression. The mother asks you to prescribe Prozac.

Discuss your management.

Issues for the patient

- Embarrassment.
- Stigma.
- Drug or alcohol misuse?
- Peer pressure, bullying?
- Attention seeking.

Issues for the doctor

- Need to assess degree of depression and risk of self-harm.
- NICE guidelines, 2004 advise GPs to treat children with mild depression in primary care.
- Initial watchful waiting for children who have 4 of the 10 symptoms of depression.
- Refer for group CBT, guided self-help or non-directive supportive therapy if symptoms persist for 4 weeks.
- Refer to a child and adolescent mental health specialist if the child fails to respond to two interventions, if depression recurs within 1 year, if child shows signs of self-neglect, or if requested by the patient or relatives.
- Refer if child has moderate-to-severe depression.
- Urgent referral to a psychiatrist if child is actively suicidal, has psychotic symptoms, exhibits severe agitation with at least seven of the symptoms of depression, or shows signs of severe self-neglect.
- Self-awareness—GP knows he/she cannot prescribe Prozac as first-line treatment for mild depression in children and therefore must explain this to the mother. Communication may be stressful if mother is adamant.
- Do no harm—inform mother that prozac is used with psychological treatments for children with moderate-to-severe depression who have not responded to psychological therapy first.
- Self-awareness—GP knows that SSRIs have been associated with increased suicidal thoughts and acts of self-harm and may have had a bad experience with a patient on SSRIs.

Issues for the mother

- End of her tether. Stressed. Guilt over depressed child. Seeking instant cure.

Issues for the practice

- Consider audit of management of depression in adolescents to assess for uniformity/equity and whether NICE guidelines are being followed.
- Consider audit of any complications with SSRIs among patients.

Question 2: Answers

Please read the extract from the paper entitled: The effectiveness of five strategies for the prevention of gastrointestinal toxicity induced by non-steroidal anti-inflammatory drugs: systematic review (please refer to **Reference material A**), and answer the question given below.

Comment on the strengths and weaknesses of the methodology of study population for this study.

Strengths

- Authors reviewed only randomised controlled trials.
- Authors used a variety of search engines.
- Exclusion criteria are listed.
- Primary and secondary outcome measures are described.
- Authors assessed trials based on whether they were truly valid (double-blinded with baseline comparability to avoid introducing confounding variables).

Weaknesses

- Primary outcomes are many and some may overlap.
- Secondary outcomes are also many and may overlap with the primary outcomes. Perhaps one or two outcomes should have been selected instead of several ranging from GI, renal, cardiac to death.
- No mention of power or confidence intervals.
- No mention of time span of treatment.
- No mention of the five strategies that the authors wish to examine.

Question 3: Answers

Forest plot Tables from the results section of the paper referred to in question 2 (The effectiveness of five strategies for the prevention of gastrointestinal toxicity induced by non-steroidal anti-inflammatory drugs: systematic review) are provided (please refer to **Reference material B**).

Interpret the results in the table.

- Proton-pump inhibitors plus non-selective NSAID *vs* placebo plus non-selective NSAID. There were only four RCTs for this group with a total of 677 participants on proton-pump inhibitors and 431 in the placebo group. Because the relative risk favoured both gastroprotector and to a small degree placebo, no conclusions can be drawn.

- Misoprostol plus non-selective NSAID *vs* placebo plus non-selective NSAID. 10 RCTs were reviewed with a total of 5780 participants in the gastroprotector group and 5727 in the placebo group. This plot shows that misoprostol reduces serious gastrointestinal complications (0.57, 0.4–0.9) as opposed to placebo. However, the result is chiefly influenced by the Silverstein 1995 study.

- Cox-2 selective NSAID *vs* non-selective NSAID. 11 RCTs were reviewed with 11,487 participants in the Cox-2 group and 9967 in the Cox-1 group. This plot shows that Cox-2 reduces serious gastrointestinal complications (90.55, 0.38–0.80) as opposed to Cox-1 drugs. The results are heavily influenced by the CLASS 2000 and Bombardier 2000 studies.

Question 4: Answers

Discuss the usefulness of the following drugs in the treatment of heart failure, giving evidence to support your views:

a) **ACE inhibitors**

Comments	Evidence
RCTs show they reduce ischaemic events, mortality, and hospital admission compared with placebo	Clinical Evidence, 2004
First-line therapy	
SOLVD study (studies of left ventricular dysfunction) showed enalapril reduced mortality in NYHA class II/III heart failure	NEJM 1991
Long-term ACE inhibitor therapy in patients with heart failure	Lancet 2000
CONSENSUS Study (Cooperative North ScandiNavian Enalapril Survival Study)	NEJM 1987
First-line therapy for newly-diagnosed HF	NICE Heart Failure Guidance

b) **Beta-blockers**

Comments	Evidence
Beta-blocker therapy in heart failure: scientific review >10,000 patients with NYHA class II-IV heart failure on beta-blockers (carvedilol, bisoprolol, metoprolol) showed reduced morbidity and mortality	*JAMA* Feb 2002
Systematic reviews show that adding a beta-blocker to an ACEI decreases mortality and hospital admission	*Clinical Evidence,* 2004
Initiating newly diagnosed HF patients on carvedilol and then adding ACEI perindopril produces greater symptom improvement. Prospective study of 78 newly diagnosed HF patients on digoxin and diuretics compared carvedilol to perindopril. The carvedilol group showed improved LV ejection fraction and plasma brain natriuretic peptide concentrations. The study is small and could be biased, as it was open labelled	*J Am Coll Cardiol* 2004;44:825–830

c) **Digoxin**

Comments	Evidence
Effect of digoxin on mortality and morbidity in patients with heart failure—showed efficacy	*NEJM* 1997
One RCT found that digoxin reduced the proportion of patients (already on diuretics and ACEI) admitted to hospital for worsening heart failure at 37 months compared with placebo, but no difference in mortality	*Clinical Evidence,* 2004

d) **Angiotensin II receptor blockers**

Comments	Evidence
One systematic review showed no difference between this drug and placebo in all-cause mortality and hospital admission in patients with NYHA Class II-IV heart failure. One possible explanation may be the small numbers of patients in the review	*Clinical Evidence,* 2004
ARB + ACEI reduces admission for heart failure compared with ACEI alone but does not reduce mortality	*Clinical Evidence,* 2004 *J Am Coll Cardiol* 2002 Feb 'ARB and ACEIs'

Question 5: Answers

Mrs Barry brings in her 4-year-old son who is small for his age. He has a history of frequent chest infections and bulky, greasy stools. You suspect cystic fibrosis.

How would you manage this patient?

Issues for the patient/mother

- Immediate concern over a sick child.
- Fear of uncertainty over child's diagnosis and prognosis.
- Fear over the management of a chronic disease.
- Fear of CF in subsequent pregnancies.
- Child may feel guilty for being different, a burden on his parents as he gets older.
- Parental fear of drainage of financial resources and energy. May lead to marital difficulties with added strain of being a carer.

Issues for the doctor

- Arrange sweat test to confirm the diagnosis.
- Arrange chest X-ray, blood for LFTs and glucose, and send stool sample for faecal fats.
- Arrange skin test for aspergillus, as 20% may develop allergic bronchopulmonary aspergillosis.
- Treat chest infections with antibiotics, ideally based on sputum culture.
- Arrange Hib, influenza, and pneumococcal vaccinations.
- Refer for a multidisciplinary approach.
- Refer to a paediatrician who specialises in CF.
- Refer to a chest physiotherapist to teach parents how to do bronchial airway drainage.
- Refer to a dietician to discuss a supplemental high-calorie diet and fat-soluble vitamins.
- Refer to a geneticist to advise on risk of CF in subsequent pregnancies (genotyping to confirm the diagnosis in the child and also the gene carrier status of the parents and relatives).
- Refer to a fertility specialist.
- Refer to a cardiothoracic surgeon if severe bronchiectasis or cor pulmonale requires heart–lung transplantation.

- Manage complications with help of multidisciplinary team—bronchiecta-sis, chest infections, cor pulmonale, diabetes (10–20%), cirrhosis, and male infertility.
- Prescribing bronchodilators, mucus-thinning drugs, pancreatic enzymes, etc on the advice of hospital specialists.
- Educate and reassure family that you are available to help them manage the child's health, that he will be under the care of several specialists working as a team, and that the prognosis is good.
- Self-awareness—doctor may not feel up-to-date with the management of CF and can use this opportunity to read up on the subject (PUNS/DENS) and consult with a paediatrician for further advice.

Question 6: Answers

Mrs Keegan brings in her 7-year-old son, Matthew, to your surgery. She reports that he wets the bed every night.

How would you manage this consultation?

Issues for Matthew

- Embarrassment, shame at wetting the bed.
- Unable to attend sleepovers with friends for fear of wetting the bed.
- ? Nightmares.
- ? Domestic stress (parents rowing, separation, divorce).
- ? Bullying at school.
- ? Too much homework or having learning difficulties.
- Low self-esteem.
- Social withdrawal.

Issues for Mrs Keegan

- Needing to change and wash the bedsheets every night.
- Lack of sleep.
- Frustration at child.
- Stress, fatigue.

Issues for the GP

- Take a history—daytime dryness, family history of bedwetting, h/o urine infections, attention-seeking behaviour, diabetes mellitus (thirst and frequent urination), diabetes insipidus (head injury, thirst, blurred vision, headache), congenital anomalies, birth anoxia, etc.
- Examine the child—growth, kidneys, abdomen for constipation, and test urine for sugar, send for MSU. Arrange renal scan to exclude congenital anomaly, e.g. bifid ureter.
- Conservative management—suggest fluid restriction, wake child at night to go to the toilet, star chart (praise dry nights), bed-wetting alarm (from enuresis clinic).
- Drug therapy if conservative management fails—desmopression spray/tablet for 3 months or imipramine.

231

- Refer child to enuresis clinic for second opinion on management.
- Refer to urology if child has UTI as unusual for boys to have UTI. Renal anomaly?

Evidence-based medicine

- According to *Clinical Evidence*, Oct 2004, one systematic review found that dry bed training had higher success rates of 14 consecutive dry nights than no treatment.
- Another review showed that enuresis alarms increase initial success rates compared with no treatment.
- Another systematic review showed that desmopressin reduces bedwetting by one night per week and increases chance of initial success (14 consecutive dry nights) compared with placebo.

Question 7: Answers

Discuss the usefulness of the following interventions for smoking cessation, giving evidence to support your views:

a) **Advice on smoking cessation**

Comments	Evidence
Systematic reviews have found that one-off advice from a physician during a routine consultation is linked with 2% of smokers quitting smoking without relapse for 1 year	*Current Evidence,* June 2004
Systematic reviews and one RCT have shown that antismoking advice improves smoking cessation in people at high risk of smoking-related diseases	*Current Evidence,* June 2004
Group or individual behavioural counselling can facilitate smoking cessation and improve quit rates	
The five 'As' for antismoking interventions: Ask about smoking at every opportunity Assess smoker's interest in stopping Advise against smoking Assist smokers to stop (set a target quit date) Arrange follow-up	Coleman T. Cessation interventions in routine health care. *BMJ* 2004 Mar;328:631–632

b) **Bupropion for smoking cessation**

Comments	Evidence
One systematic review showed that bupropion increases quit rates at 1 year	*Current Evidence, June 2004*
NICE approves bupropion (Zyban) on the NHS. Bupropion is a monocyclic antidepressant structurally related to amphetamine. Zyban is a sustained-release formulation of bupropion HCl	NICE
Bupropion had a 1-year cessation rate 13% higher than placebo in one trial	*Prescrire Int'l France*
However, in the initial 6 months of use in Ireland, there were 12 overdose cases which resulted in tachycardia, drowsiness, fits, and cardiac arrhythmias	Bupropion toxicity. *Irish Med J*, Jan 2002

c) **Nicotine replacement therapy for smoking cessation**

Comments	Evidence
One systematic review and one RCT showed that NRT is an effective adjunct to cessation strategies in smokers who smoke at least 10 cigs a day. However, three RCTs showed that the benefit of NRT on quit rates reduced with time	*Current Evidence*, June 2004
NRT yields a 1-year cessation rate of 14–18% vs 10% with placebo	*Prescrire Int'l France*, Dec 2001
Prescriptions for NRT cost £20–56 million annually compared to the cost of treating smoking-related diseases (£150 million). GPs should prescribe using the abstinent-contingent protocol	NICE
Use of transdermal nicotine patches over 12 weeks is very cost-effective and doubles the success rate of brief advice at 1 year	

Question 8: Answers

Discuss how you would develop a practice protocol for diabetic care.

Aims

- Practice meeting to discuss and decide on aims of this practice protocol. Ensure all relevant health-care professionals are present.

Background

- Research current guidelines. QOF targets in diabetes of HbA$_{1C}$ <7.4 and BP <145/85 mm Hg.
- UKPDS suggests lowering BP reduces incidence of MI and CVA by 44%.
- Need for annual ophthalmology review, neurological checks, chiropody. Need to check fasting lipids. Need to advise on weight, diet, and taking up exercise. Need to offer flu and pneumococcal vaccinations.

Target groups

- Screening.
- Diet-controlled diabetics and impaired glucose tolerance.
- NIDDM.
- IDDM.

Funding

- To involve pharma companies?
- Offer proposal to PCT for funding.

Follow-up

- Decide on intervals of follow-up of diabetic patients.
- Will this be shared hospital and GP care or primarily GP-based? Establish exclusion criteria.
- Coordinate and liaise with secondary services for optimum diabetic care.

Audit

- Of current practice to identify areas of improvement.
- Offer diabetic patients satisfaction survey to assess current practice.
- Need to re-audit after change has been implemented. Set time limit.

Responsibility

- Decide who will be the lead person for accountability when things go wrong or right, a person to lead SEA if needed.

Refer

- Establish criteria for when patients need to be referred to hospital for outpatient care or emergency treatment.

Review and update

- Decide how often the protocol will be reviewed and updated.

Question 9: Answers

Mr Santos holds you hostage in your room. He demands a sick note from you for his probation officer and tells you that he will go to jail if you do not issue one. He raises his voice and stands above you menacingly.

What do you do? What issues does this raise?

Issues for the patient

- Use of aggression to manipulate the doctor or other people in his life.
- Is his aggression due to alcohol or drug misuse or is this cultural?
- Has he a prior history of intimidating staff? Is he on probation for ABH or GBH?

Issues for the doctor

- Immediate concern for personal safety.
- Assess room layout and whether patient is blocking exit.
- Locate and press the panic button.
- Use nonverbal and verbal means of communication to diffuse the situation. Remain seated with body turned sideways to appear less confrontational. Lower pitch of voice and speak softly.
- Use negotiating and communication skills to try to come to a mutual understanding but do not accept blackmail.
- Document everything. Log in incident book for SEA.
- Need for practice meeting to decide whether patient's behaviour warrants a warning or immediate deduction.
- Need to contact the police for an incident number if partners deem that patient should be removed. Then inform PCT or 7-day rule will apply and patient will still be entitled to medical care.
- Neighbour's housekeeping—able to see next patient? Debrief with colleague. Time out. Inform patients of a delay.
- Self-awareness—feelings of panic, stress, loss of control, PTSD.

Issues for the practice

- Health and Safety at the Workplace ensures staff's right to safety at work and highlights assessment of risk.

- Practice meeting to discuss whether practice should adopt the NHS's 1999 zero tolerance policy.
- Significant events analysis—record, analyse, and review.
- Security—invest in CCTV, personal alarms, etc.
- Training of staff in dealing with violent patients. Invite speaker from Suzy Lamplugh Trust or local police officer.
- Rearrange consulting rooms so that patient cannot impede the exit.

Wider issues

- MDU survey showed that 23% of 1044 respondents had been physically assaulted over the last 5 years.
- Fear of violence may lead to a shortage of GPs in particular inner city deprived areas.

Question 10: Answers

Discuss the usefulness of the following interventions for secondary prevention of ischaemic heart events, citing evidence to support your views:

a) **Advice on lifestyle**

Comments	Evidence
One systematic review showed that cardiac rehabilitation using exercise reduces risk	*Clinical Evidence,* June 2004
There were no RCTs on the effects of smoking cessation on reducing cardiovascular events in people with coronary heart disease	*Clinical Evidence,* June 2004
Low-fat diets are of unknown effectiveness	*Clinical Evidence,* June 2004
Eating oily fish has been shown to reduce mortality at 2 years. Another RCT showed that fish oil capsules reduced mortality at 3.5 years	*Clinical Evidence,* June 2004
One systematic review of RCTs showed that stress management may decrease rates of MI in patients with coronary heart disease	*Clinical Evidence,* June 2004
Systematic reviews and large RCTs showed that lowering cholesterol in patients at high risk of ischaemic heart disease substantially reduces all-cause mortality, coronary mortality, and non-fatal MI	*Current Evidence,* June 2004
Reducing cholesterol levels by 30% reduced mortality	4S Study. *Lancet* 1994;344:1383–1389

b) **Aspirin**

Comments	Evidence
One systematic review showed that prolonged use of aspirin 75–150 mg daily is as effective as high doses	*Clinical Evidence*, June 2004
25% reduction in vascular events with aspirin (75–325 mg) in secondary prevention	Antiplatelet Trialists' Collaboration. Overview of randomised trials of antiplatelets. *BMJ* 1994;308:81–106
Aspirin shown to reduce vascular events	ISIS 2 trial

c) **Beta-blockers**

Comments	Evidence
Systematic reviews in patients post-MI showed that long-term beta-blockers reduce all-cause mortality, coronary mortality, recurrent non-fatal MI, and sudden death	*Current Evidence*, June 2004
Benefit of beta-blockers with reduction in mortality, recurrent MI and sudden death	ISIS 1 trial

d) **ACE inhibitors**

Comments	Evidence
Patients with heart failure or low ejection fraction benefit most from ACEI, with reduction in mortality	ISIS 4
Patients with ejection fractions of <40% benefited from captopril	SAVE (Survival and Ventricular Enlargement) study
One large RCT showed that in high-risk patients with LV dysfunction ramipril reduces the combined outcome of CV death, CVA, and MI *vs* placebo after 5 years	
One systematic review showed that in patients post MI with LV dysfunction, ACEI reduces mortality, hospital admission for CHF, and recurrent non-fatal MI *vs* placebo after 2 years	*Clinical Evidence*, June 2004

Question 11: Answers

Mrs Charlotte Winter brings in her toddler, Louisa, to your surgery. She states that she thinks that Louisa is allergic to peanuts.

What do you do?

Issues for Louisa

- Oral exposure to peanuts?
- Transcutaneous absorption from skin creams or oils containing peanut oil?
- Exposure *in utero* or through breast milk?
- 90% of peanut allergy sufferers have other allergies.
- Risk factors—eczema, use of soya milk formulas during infancy.
- Life-long allergy for most. 20% will outgrow sensitivity.
- Death from anaphylaxis in children is chiefly through asphyxia from laryngeal oedema and severe bronchospasm.

Issues for the mother

- Fear that Louisa will inadvertently be exposed to peanuts or crude peanut oil and die from anaphylactic shock.
- Need for reassurance and education on the management of peanut allergy.

Issues for the doctor

- 1–2% of UK children are allergic to peanuts.
- Obtain a careful history from mother and perform an examination of Louisa.
- If she has indeed had an allergic response to peanuts, refer Louisa to hospital paediatric allergy specialist for oral challenge test and measure of IgE to confirm the diagnosis.
- Is there a family history of peanut allergy? Higher prevalence.
- Advise mother of potential cross-reactivity to other nuts/legumes—tree nuts and in rare cases, beans, peas, and soy.
- Educate mother on how to manage peanut allergy.
- Prescribe preloaded syringes or autoinjectors containing a single dose of

0.15 mg epinephrine (Epipen Junior, Anapen Junior) for children between 15 and 30 kg. Inform mother that the dose may be repeated after 10–15 min as necessary. Decide on a clear emergency treatment plan with mother for inadvertent exposure. May have practice nurse teach mother how to administer intramuscular injections.

- Inform nursery workers of Louisa's allergy, have an emergency kit at the daycare centre, and ensure teachers are instructed on its use.
- Suggest that Mrs Winter contacts the Anaphylaxis Campaign, Medic Alert Foundation, and Allergy UK for further advice and support.

Question 12: Answers

Comment on the following, citing evidence to support your views:

a) **Benefit of patient-centred consultations**

Comments	Evidence
Patients who received less explanation were less satisfied and less compliant	Francis, 1969
Video-recorded consultations improved patient-centredness but led to increased length of consultations	Verby, 1979
Comparison of two practices conducting 5- or 10-min consultations showed that fewer prescriptions were issued and return consultations halved within the following 4 weeks. Referral rates and diagnoses were similar	Hughes, 1983
Developed 'ICE'—exploring the patients' ideas, concerns, and expectations	Pendleton, 1980s
Comparison of older male GPs to younger female GPs showed that female GPs had longer consultations and greater job satisfaction	Calnan, 1988
Longer patient-centred consultations led to increased GP stress. There was more patient satisfaction but no difference in referral rates or return consultations	Howie, 1992

b) **Heartsink patients and communication skills**

Comments	Evidence
May be a problem of doctor–patient communication and not being able to come to a mutual understanding at the end of a consultation	Butler and Evans BJGP, 1999;Mar:230
Number of heartsink patients is directly proportional to doctor's poor communication skills. Suggest smaller lists, reducing workload, longer consultations, and more time out to attend courses	Mathers BJGP, 1995;45:293